THE
INFLAMMATORY
RESET

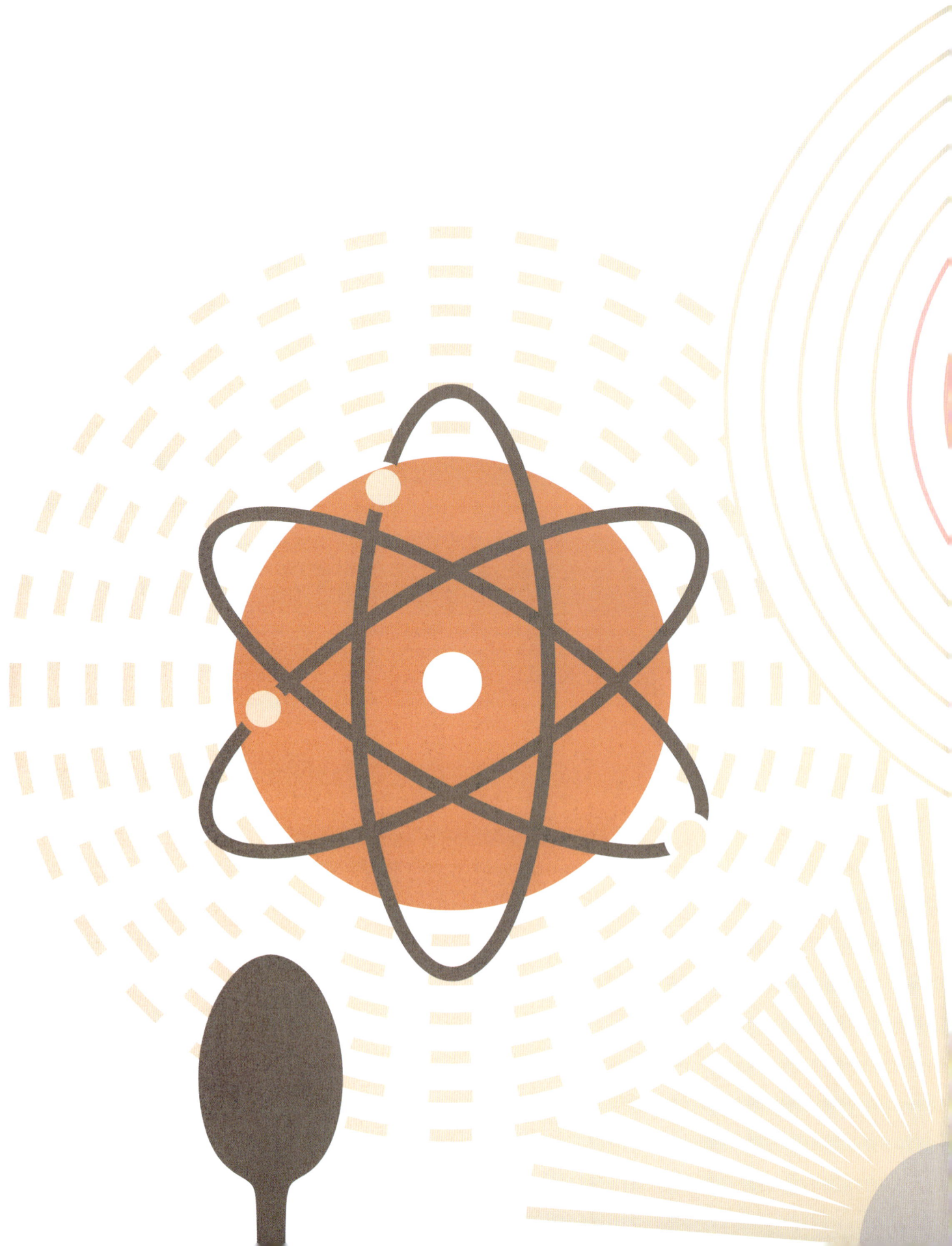

THE INFLAMMATORY RESET

YOUR GUIDE TO REDUCING INFLAMMATION

DR. JOSH REDD WITH **KARALYNNE CALL**

Copyright © 2024 Dr. Josh Redd

All rights reserved. No part of this publication may be reproduced, distributed, or transmitted in any form or by any means, including photocopying, recording, or other electronic or mechanical methods, without the prior written permission of the publisher, except in the case of brief quotations embodied in critical reviews and certain other noncommercial uses permitted by copyright law. For permission requests, write to the publisher, addressed "Attention: Permissions Coordinator," at the address below.

PalmaVita Books, LLC
10965 S River Front Pkwy
South Jordan, UT 84095

ISBN: 979-8-9884544-0-3 (hardcover)
Library of Congress Control Number: 2023917583

Design by *the*BookDesigners
First printing edition 2024

Printed in China

While the facts I provide in this book are based on general knowledge and the success stories I have personally seen in my clinics, the information contained in this book is for informational purposes only and should not be taken as medical advice. I do not provide personalized medical advice through publications such as this book. You should consult your doctor or qualified medical personnel for personalized advice before making any changes to your diet or taking any supplements. If you are having a medical emergency or urgent health concern, do not rely on the information provided in this book, as personalized medical care might be needed. Please seek medical attention or call local emergency services. Any third-party information or materials mentioned in this book are included only to provide the reader with additional sources for review. I am not responsible for the content, accuracy, or privacy practices of these third-party publications.

Introduction 1
How to Use This Book 3

PART ONE: INFLAMMATION & WHY IT MATTERS 5

1. What Is Inflammation? 6
2. How Can Inflammation Affect You? 7
   a. Brain, Cognition, & Inflammation 7
   b. Gut Health 8
   c. Hormone Imbalances 9
   d. Liver & Gallbladder 9
   e. Weight Gain & Inflammation 10
   f. Blood Sugar Crashes 10
   g. Raising Cholesterol Levels 11
   h. Heart Disease 11
   i. Autoimmune Diseases 11
3. Causes of Inflammation 12
   a. Dietary Roots in Inflammation 12
   b. Inflammatory Lifestyles 13
   c. Neurology & Inflammation 14
   d. Emotional Causes of Inflammation 15
   e. Cortisol, Estrogen, Insulin, & Inflammation 15
4. Environmental Toxins & How to Buffer Them 18
   a. BPA & BPS 19
   b. Dioxins 20
   c. Parabens 21
   d. Phthalates 23
   e. PFAS (Perfluoroalkyl & Polyfluoroalkyl Substances) 24
   f. Glyphosate 25
   g. Flame Retardants 26
5. Covid & Inflammation 28

PART TWO: THE INFLAMMATORY RESET ... 31

1. The Inflammatory Reset ... 32
2. Activities & Exercises to Reduce Inflammation ... 33
   a. A Lifestyle to Reduce Inflammation ... 33
   b. Exercise ... 34
   c. Meditation ... 35
   d. Stimulating the Vagus Nerve ... 36
   e. Ice Baths & Cold Showers ... 36
   f. Infrared Sauna ... 37
   g. Alpha-Stim Training ... 37
   h. Hyperbaric Oxygen Therapy ... 38
3. Resetting Your Diet ... 39
   a. Foods to Avoid ... 40
   b. Foods to Eat ... 41
4. Reintroducing Eliminated Foods ... 42
5. Supplements & Inflammation ... 43
6. Sample Protocol ... 46
7. Fasting While on the Inflammatory Reset ... 47
   a. The Benefits of Fasting with Inflammation ... 47
   b. When You Should Not Fast ... 48
8. Small Intestinal Bacterial Overgrowth (SIBO) ... 49
9. Resetting for 90 Days ... 49

PART THREE: RECIPES ... 51

1. Breakfast ... 55
2. Drinks & Smoothies ... 75
3. Sides, Snacks, & Salads ... 89
4. Main Dishes ... 112
5. Soups & Stews ... 139

About Our Recipe Developer & Photographer 155
You Can Do It 157

APPENDICES 159

1. **Cutting-Edge Testing** 160
2. **Inflammatory-Focused Clinics** 162
3. **Recommended Products & Tools** 164
   a. Air & Water 164
   b. Kitchen & Cookware 164
   c. Gardening 165
   d. Skin Care, Cosmetics, & Body Applicators 166
   e. Equipment for Anti-Inflammatory Exercises 166
   f. Food & Nutrition 167
   g. Dietary Supplements 167
4. **Endnotes** 169

About the Authors 204

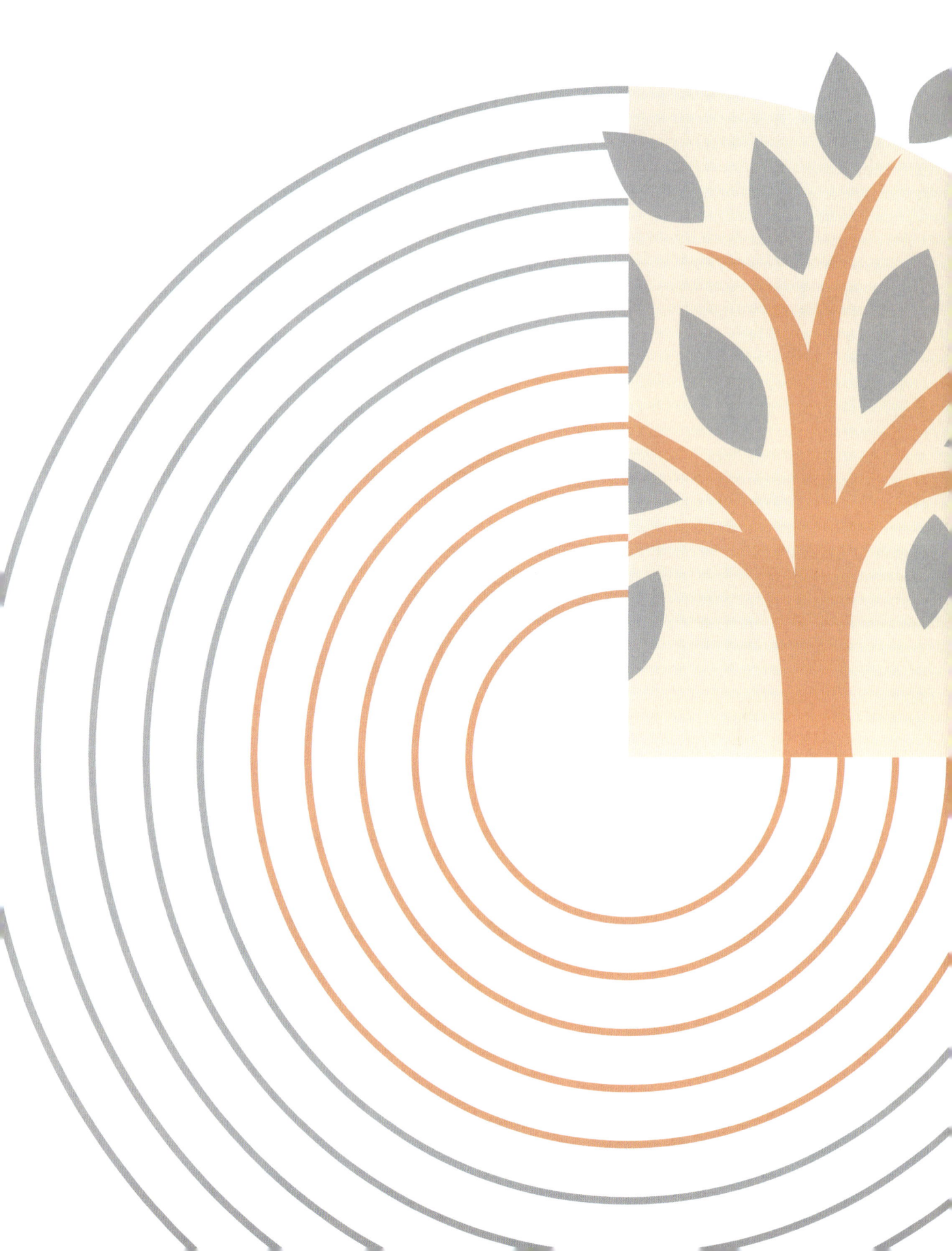

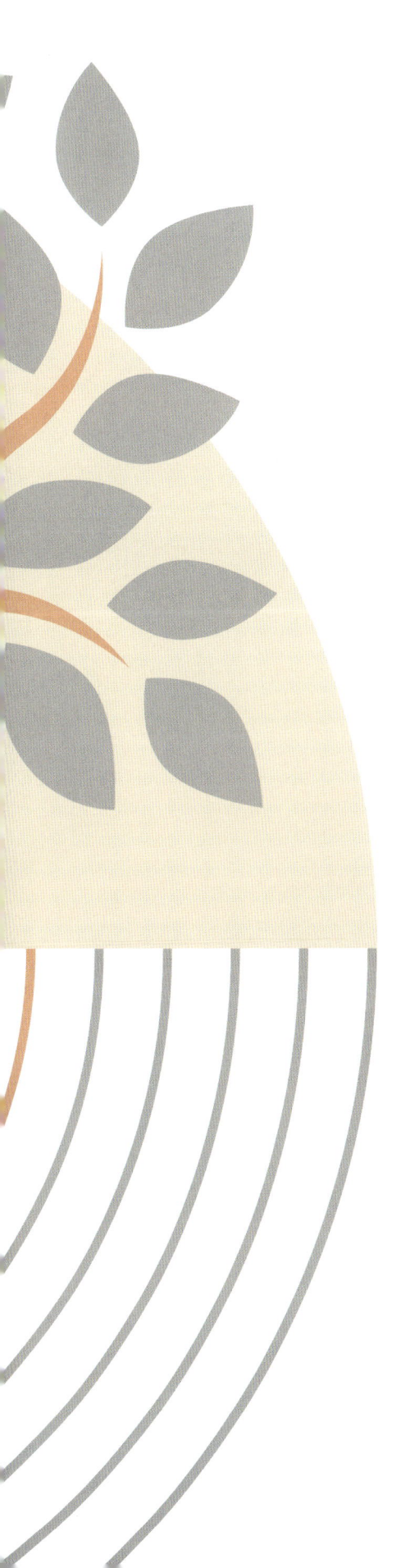

INTRODUCTION

If you are reading this book, chances are that you or your loved ones are dealing with symptoms or health issues from inflammation. The inflammation crisis in this country is causing a spike in chronic health conditions and impacting countless lives.

We all live inflammatory lifestyles, though we might not realize it. We are overly stressed, our food is overly processed and full of sugar, and we are constantly exposed to environmental irritants that can trigger inflammatory pathways, largely unaware of their unavoidable impact on our health. Inflammation underlies most chronic diseases today, from diabetes to thyroid issues to Alzheimer's, and causes issues such as fatigue, depression, hormonal difficulties, chronic pain, gut problems, and so on. Just about every health disorder these days can be traced to inflammation. While dampening inflammation lowers disease risk, a bigger reason to tackle it is because it gives you your life back.

The Inflammatory Reset is a 30-day program to help you take control of your inflammation. My goal with this program is to allow you to understand what inflammation is, why most of us have it now, and simple strategies—exercises, lifestyle changes, and a diet—that will dramatically reduce your inflammation in a month. If you follow these strategies, you, your kids, or your loved ones will feel substantial improvements to your health in that time. Imagine your life with things such as better digestion, more energy, and clearer thinking. This is your guidebook to put the power of improving your health back into your hands. Doctors like myself are great secondary tools to consult on your journey; we are available to serve, lift, comfort,

THE INFLAMMATORY RESET

and, most importantly, educate and empower. Bottom line, you decide what's best for your health. With this guide, you'll have the autonomy of improving the quality of your own life through exercise, behaviors, and diet.

HOW TO USE THIS BOOK

This book does a few things. It not only provides information on the kinds of inflammation and what it does to the body, but also offers easy action steps to reduce it and a whole slew of great recipes that can keep you honest and consistent. I'd recommend reading this book once all the way through. Heck, we put a lot of time into it, but I'm sure even the inflammation veteran will find a gem or a learning point to challenge the way you think about inflammation and how you can reduce it.

I designed this book to be a resource, and a resource for everyone. Maybe you're here because you think you have inflammation and you're looking for descriptions of symptoms in the next chapter or further resources in the appendix. Maybe a loved one suffers from inflammation and, while they're not the most food-savvy, you can help them prepare some of the delicious recipes in this book that will help them feel better and continue to enjoy the foods they love. We're all at different points in our journeys to treat inflammation, and you can pick up this book as a reference that you can use over and over to improve the quality of life for yourself or loved ones.

As I mentioned in the introduction, this book is about learning and empowerment, and *The Inflammatory Reset* is meant to be used more than once and something you can go back to when you feel you need it.

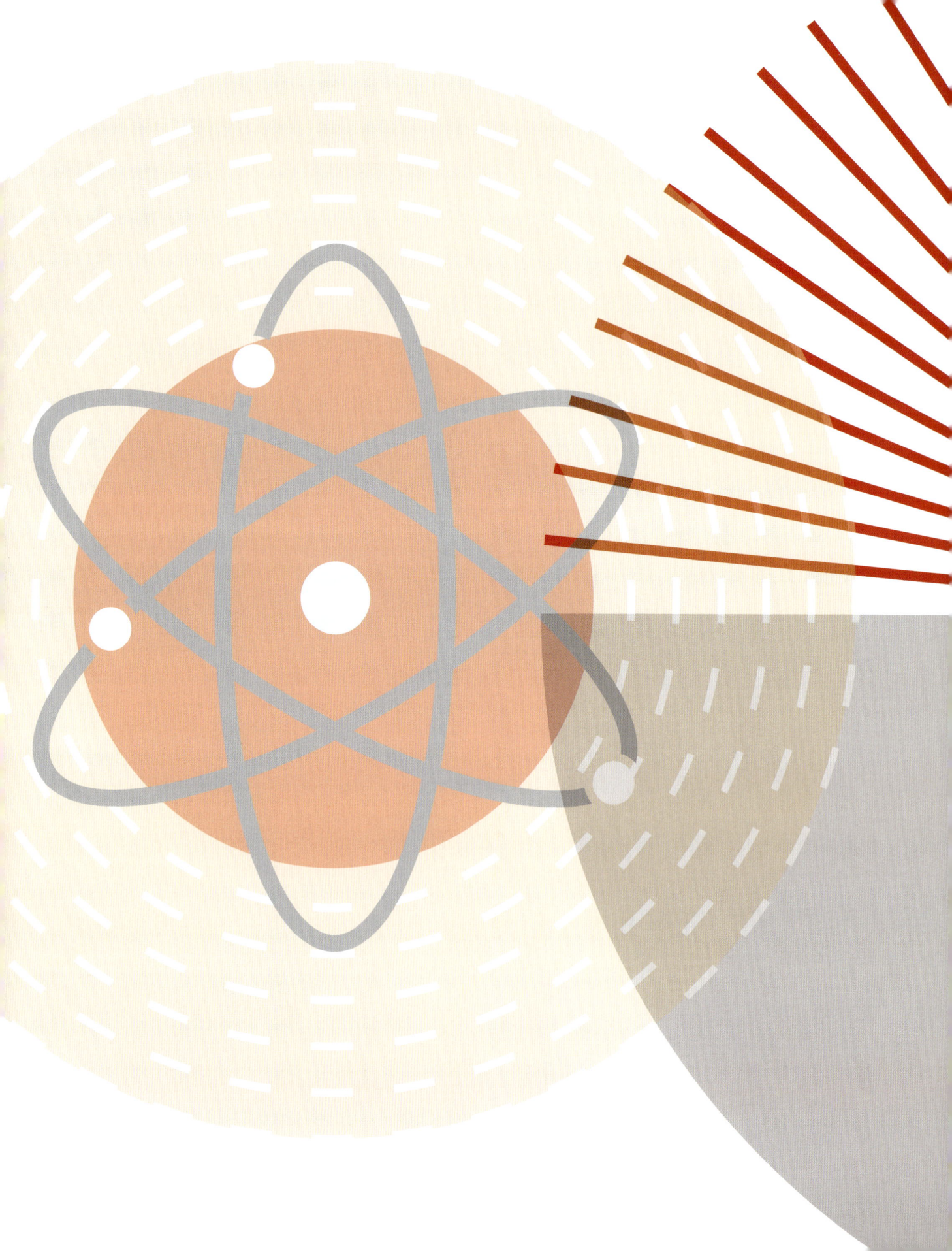

PART ONE

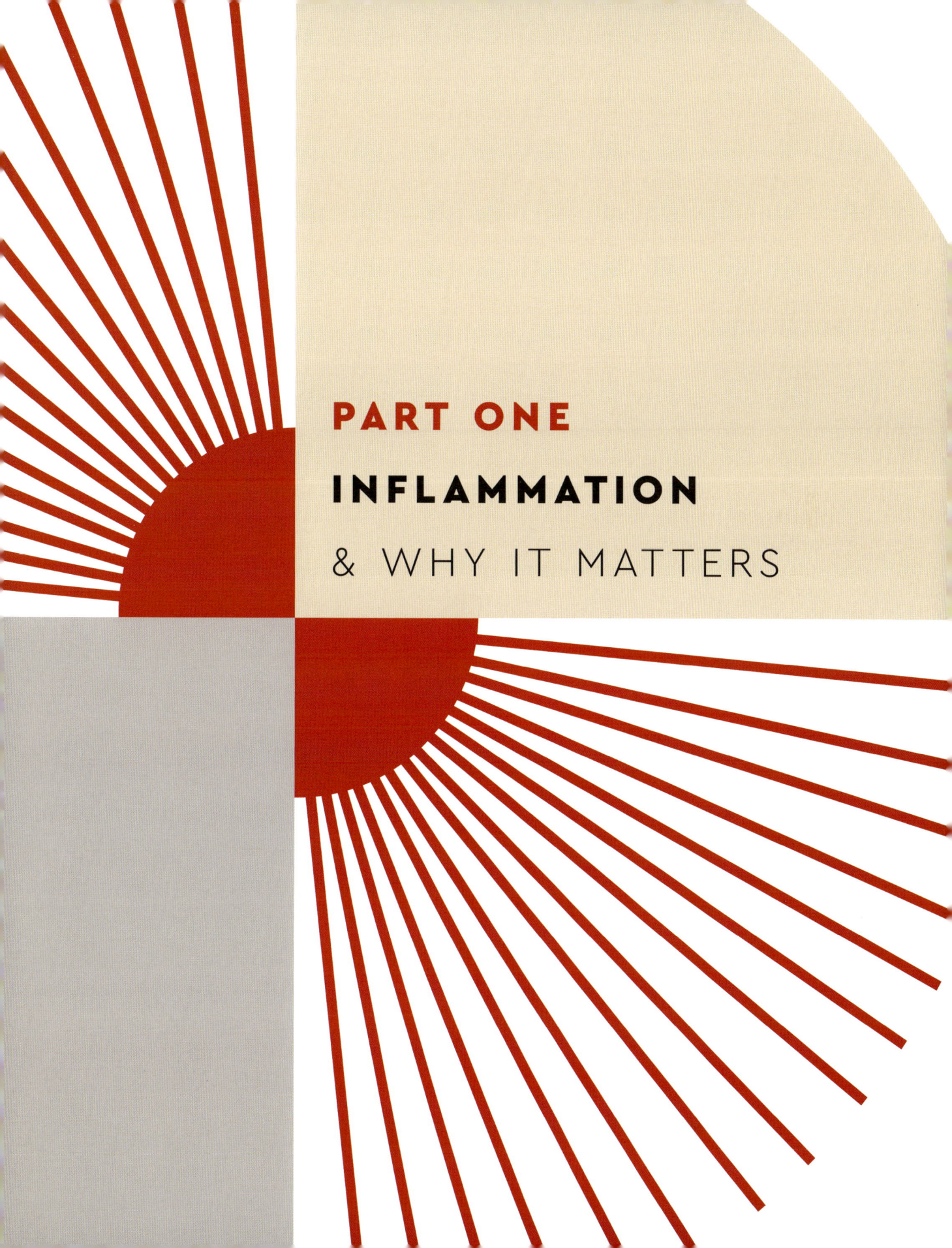

INFLAMMATION

& WHY IT MATTERS

WHAT IS INFLAMMATION?

Inflammation is directly tied to the immune system and acts as a protective physiological response. Our cells are hardwired with **pattern recognition receptors** and a variety of other blockades that alert our immune system to the threat of a virus, environmental irritants, cells damaged by injury or inflammation, or anything harmful that it doesn't recognize. This response ignites different inflammatory mediators or pathways to combat whatever triggered it. As a short-term response, this is fantastic. This is **acute inflammation**, and it keeps us healthy and out of danger.

But when these inflammatory pathways are triggered frequently—and without outside danger—they can aggravate and destroy surrounding tissues, creating even more inflammation. This is **chronic inflammation**, and it can create a vicious cycle that sets off a litany of other diseases. Though chronic inflammation can be difficult to combat if you don't know what's going on, taking the steps I've laid out for you in *The Inflammatory Reset* will give you the tools to spot inflammation when it arises in your body.

HOW CAN INFLAMMATION AFFECT YOU?

As I mentioned, there is an inflammation crisis in this country. From our workload to our diet to our environment, inflammatory triggers are pervasive in our lifestyles and lead to a medley of chronic health conditions. Studies show chronic inflammation and the factors that contribute to it—particularly high blood sugar and insulin resistance—underlie the most common health disorders and diseases today.

The kinds of inflammation your body can experience may seem overwhelming, but I want to show how commonplace inflammation is and what symptoms the Inflammatory Reset can alleviate or even heal in your body.

BRAIN, COGNITION, & INFLAMMATION

While short bouts of inflammation clean up the brain so we have healthy synapses firing, chronic inflammation reduces all neurotransmitter conduction. One of the most common symptoms is brain fog. If you feel overly fatigued after reading a book or driving long distances—or just feel like you live with brain fog—that could be a sign of inflammation in your brain.

Other brain-based symptoms of inflammation can include depression, low motivation, memory loss, clumsiness, and irritability. What's worse, these symptoms indicate your brain may be aging too fast, putting you at a higher risk for brain-degenerative diseases such as dementia and Alzheimer's.

Additionally, brain inflammation can lead to other kinds of inflammation down the line. Our clinics see patients from the NFL and MLS with serious concussions that have led to various health issues, ranging from gastrointestinal disorders to autoimmune disease and cardiovascular disease. The good news is that through diet and lifestyle modifications, we can begin reversing brain inflammation. As you progress through the Inflammatory Reset, you can look forward to less brain fog, better focus, more energy, and an overall enhanced sense of well-being.

THE INFLAMMATORY RESET

GUT HEALTH

Chronic inflammation promotes intestinal permeability, also known as leaky gut, where undigested food proteins pass from inside the gastrointestinal tract through the cells that line the gut wall and into the rest of the body. This increases the likelihood of gut infections, gut inflammation, food intolerances, and other gut issues. Leaky gut produces many symptoms, but these are some of the more common ones I've seen in my practice:

- Gas
- Bloating
- Loose stools
- IBS
- Yeast overgrowth
- SIBO (small intestinal bacterial overgrowth)
- Food intolerances and sensitivities
- Seasonal allergies
- Chronic skin problems like acne, eczema, and rashes
- Mood dysregulation
- Issues with concentration and memory

In terms of stomach health, we are conditioned to think that acid is bad and the cause of both heartburn and acid reflux. But sufficient stomach acid actually *prevents* acid reflux in most cases and is vital to healthy gut and immune function. Inflammation may inhibit the production of stomach acid, and low stomach acid, or hypochlorhydria, can cause numerous gut disorders as well as poor protein absorption. The most common disorder we see as a result of low stomach acid is gastroesophageal reflux disease (GERD). These are some of the symptoms associated with GERD:

- Heartburn
- Regurgitation
- Chronic cough
- Chest pain
- Dysphagia (difficulty swallowing)

Chronic inflammation in the digestive tract, which extends from the stomach all the way down to the colon, increases the likelihood of gut infections, gut inflammation, food intolerance, GERD, and all of the other symptoms I have listed thus far. Implementing the Inflammatory Reset to restore balance to your digestive system is pivotal in bringing your body into a state of homeostasis. Your gut wants to be repaired, and the body has tremendous potential to heal, more than we were ever taught. The Inflammatory Reset will help you heal your leaky gut, reduce systemic inflammation, experience better sleep, decrease stress, and gain more energy.

HORMONE IMBALANCES

In women, high inflammation is associated with symptoms that range from hair loss, infertility, and complications in childbirth to an increased risk of autism, allergies, and other health challenges in their offspring. Women who experience symptoms of dysregulated hormones as a result of high systemic inflammation also are at risk of experiencing a more difficult transition from perimenopause to menopause. Reducing inflammation through diet and lifestyle can also reduce hormone-related conditions like polycystic ovary syndrome (PCOS), premenstrual syndrome (PMS), infertility, and perimenopausal and menopausal symptoms like vaginal dryness, hot flashes, weight gain, and low libido.

LIVER & GALLBLADDER

Your liver and gallbladder are vital organs for healthy digestion and detoxification. Inflammation causes both to become sluggish and contributes to gallstones in the gallbladder. When these organs aren't at proper functional levels, their ability to clear toxins and metabolized hormones is hampered, increasing the overall toxicity in your body, which can lead to its own set of problems, including hormonal imbalances, infertility, and weight loss resistance.

Shifting into a more anti-inflammatory lifestyle—by cleaning up your diet or detoxing household items and cosmetic products—automatically supports your liver. The job of the liver is detoxification, so anything you can do to make that organ's job easier will have a profound impact on your health.

WEIGHT GAIN & INFLAMMATION

Weight gain and weight loss resistance are often problematic issues for people with chronic inflammation. That's because inflammation slows down metabolism, shuts down cellular receptor sites for fat-burning hormones, and stalls muscle building.

Resistance to weight loss can be incredibly frustrating, but understanding that inflammation is often at the root of the problem provides a key to a door that we previously felt was locked. With inflammation under control, and along with a whole foods diet that minimizes carbohydrates, your body can return to its normal level of metabolizing food and burning fat. Practicing the Inflammatory Reset's diet will not only lower your inflammation but also challenge you to eat healthier foods and help you manage your weight.

BLOOD SUGAR CRASHES

Inflammation causes slow uptake, poor utilization, and inefficient elimination of glucose by the cells, all of which makes people more prone to blood sugar crashes. Symptoms can include brain fog, irritability, lightheadedness, and adrenal fatigue. During the 30 days of your Inflammatory Reset, you can expect your glucose numbers to trend down, resulting in steadier blood sugar levels. It's important to stick to your new diet long-term, though, as reversing insulin resistance often takes longer than a month.

RAISING CHOLESTEROL LEVELS

Because inflammation causes you to store fat more quickly than it's burned, it can cause unhealthy cholesterol markers. These include high triglycerides, high cholesterol, and small, dense LDL ("bad") cholesterol. In turn, high cholesterol can lead to fatty deposits in your blood cells and increase your risk of heart disease.

With the Inflammatory Reset, you can rebalance your cholesterol levels and reduce your risk of heart disease. For some people this can happen in a month or two; for others it takes longer, depending on how long they have been dealing with inflammation, high cholesterol, and other health factors.

HEART DISEASE

Inflammation is now recognized as a primary cause of heart disease. This is because it can lead to high levels of the amino acid homocysteine, which increases the risk of heart disease, dementia, and other neurodegenerative diseases. Inflammation is also associated with insulin resistance, elevated blood sugar, dysfunction in the lining of the blood vessels, increased blood pressure, and declining brain function—all of which contribute to cardiovascular disease.

Just like with high cholesterol, reducing systemic inflammation is one of the fastest ways to reduce your risk of heart disease. The Inflammatory Reset is a lifeline that can enable you to take control of your heart health.

AUTOIMMUNE DISEASES

Autoimmunity stems from an immune system that has become overzealous, inflamed, and imbalanced. Once you develop one autoimmune disease, you're at an increased risk for developing more. You actually might already have another autoimmune reaction happening, it's just not advanced enough to produce symptoms yet.

Lowering inflammation reduces your risk of autoimmune diseases by simply altering your internal and external environment to a state that is less prone to the development of autoimmune conditions. And, if you already have been diagnosed with an autoimmune condition, lowering inflammation is the first step you can take to get your disease into remission.

CAUSES OF INFLAMMATION

While everyone has different triggers, the primary causes of inflammation typically fall into five major categories: dietary, lifestyle, physiological, neurological, and emotional. A lot of these are intertwined, not unlike the body itself: if you have one of these issues, you may have another one or two.

In learning about the causes of your inflammation, you have a better chance of lessening its toll on your body and resetting your health to previous and optimal levels.

DIETARY ROOTS IN INFLAMMATION

In the US, most of our food isn't real food anymore. Large quantities of the foods sold in our stores are ultra-processed and filled with synthetic materials. I strongly encourage you to look at labels on some of the foods you buy. If an ingredient doesn't sound natural, it's probably not good for you and could be a part of your inflammation.

Remember our pattern recognition receptors and the other immune blockades I talked about? The ones that can be triggered if they detect a foreign agent? Our immune system isn't dumb. In fact, it has been genetically programmed for thousands of years to recognize whether something is foreign or not. If we eat highly processed foods that contain a lot of synthetic material, our immune system will eventually throw its arms up in frustration.

The processed carbohydrates common in processed foods increase blood sugar, thus promoting inflammation and disease. Processed foods are also loaded with gluten, which is linked to at least 55 diseases, most of them autoimmune. While people are more aware of gluten allergies and intolerances today, most people aren't aware they have an intolerance or even have celiac disease, both of which are ubiquitous among people with chronic inflammation.

CAUSES OF INFLAMMATION

The brain consists primarily of fat, and the fats you consume determine your brain's health. Industrialized seed oils and hydrogenated oils—staple ingredients in processed foods—have been shown to boost inflammation and lead to obesity, diabetes, and brain degeneration. These oils are very high in omega-6 fatty acids, which also cause inflammation and promote chronic disease.

Humans need a balance between omega-6 and omega-3 fatty acids. Over-processed foods have a higher imbalance—more omega-6s—so seeking out foods high in omega-3s, such as salmon, chia seeds, and walnuts, is a great way to restore this balance and give your body the healthy fats it needs.

INFLAMMATORY LIFESTYLES

Being overly sedentary, sleeping poorly, and chronic stress can all lead to inflammation. Exercise combats inflammation from sedentary lifestyles effectively and can even help you sleep better. We spend a third of our days sleeping, and getting good sleep is very important to how our body functions on all fronts. Inflammation affects the sleep centers of the brain and shortens the sleep cycles necessary for growth and repair. Also, people with chronic inflammation often deal with chronic pain, robbing them of restful sleep, which becomes a vicious cycle as adequate sleep is vital to dampening inflammation.

Stress can be hard to manage. Things like a bad relationship or a toxic workplace can keep you in a state of chronic stress, thereby raising inflammation. Your mental health is important, and I recommend seeking therapy or counseling to help you pinpoint the roots of chronic stress. Managing your lifestyle is about more than your diet, and you must address all contributing factors to reset your inflammation.

NEUROLOGY & INFLAMMATION

Head trauma, addiction to drugs, and too much light from screen time can all cause brain inflammation. Your brain is your most important asset in your body, and seeking remedies for neurological inflammation should be done sooner than later. Whether you seek out medical assistance for head injuries, get help for addiction, or even change the color settings on your monitor to night mode to reduce eyestrain, you're off to a great start to reset your inflammation.

Other common causes for neurological inflammation include food intolerances—particularly to gluten and dairy—along with gut inflammation, hormonal imbalances, unmanaged autoimmune disease, and a leaky blood-brain barrier. The most common symptoms of brain inflammation are brain fog, slowed and/or fuzzy thinking, fatigue, and depression. If you constantly feel these symptoms, consider seeing a doctor for neurological inflammation.

A WORD ON ALCOHOL

It's common knowledge that alcohol isn't the best for your brain and memory. And in regard to inflammation, a hangover is a literal swelling of the brain. This may be easy to shrug off, but more research is constantly coming out to reveal the growing detriments of alcohol to your health. Initially, it was thought that only chronic and heavy alcohol use caused damage to your brain cells. However, new research shows that even moderate amounts of alcohol over an extended period can damage these cells.

The science behind this can get dense, but essentially there are two major kinds of cells at play here: **neurons**, the fundamental brain units, and **glial cells**, the protectors and brain cleaners. As neurons and glial cells die, brain mass starts to degenerate. The rapid destruction of neurons leads not only to impaired decision making, mood, and behavior but also to neurodegeneration and neurodegenerative diseases such as dementia. In fact, the second leading cause of dementia is alcoholic dementia. Depending on your source, alcohol accounts for 1–10% of the dementia cases in the United States.

Now, I'm not going to tell you to not enjoy a glass of wine with dinner, but I am asking you to consider the newest research on alcohol and inflammation. You have a finite number of neurons, and continuous drinking can lead to inflammatory conditions in your brain that will be detrimental to your health in the long term.

EMOTIONAL CAUSES OF INFLAMMATION

Did you know experiences from childhood can provoke your inflammation? Abuse, neglect, grief, and other childhood traumas can unfortunately become a lifelong "operating system" that triggers ongoing inflammation. Also, toxic relationships that you are in now can affect your mental health and increase chronic inflammation.

This kind of chronic and unpredictable stress constantly floods the body with stress hormones to keep it in a hypervigilant and inflammatory state. It's a defense mechanism in overdrive that, in time, interferes with the body's ability to turn off or dampen the stress response.

Although childhood trauma can increase inflammation and risk of disease in adulthood, your brain and body have the capacity to change. Many therapeutic methods have been shown to help heal these traumas: meditation, mindfulness practices, neurofeedback, EMDR (eye movement desensitization and reprocessing) therapy, cognitive therapy, EFT (emotional freedom technique, or tapping), therapeutic tremoring, prayer, and more. Additionally, psilocybin-guided therapy, ketamine treatments, and ayahuasca treatments, while not universally legal, have shown incredible outcomes in studies, including improving neural pathways. As I mentioned earlier, seeking help is always a great option. Therapists and various kinds of counselors can help you discover and heal stress points.

Be sure to include your emotional well-being and the health of your operating system, which was established in childhood, in your Inflammatory Reset.

CORTISOL, ESTROGEN, INSULIN & INFLAMMATION

In our practice, we see a number of triggers that drive inflammation, but three physiological factors in particular often work together to substantially increase inflammation and autoimmune flares: cortisol, estrogen, and insulin.

CORTISOL

Cortisol is an adrenal hormone that governs our stress responses. People with chronic inflammation often have cortisol levels that are chronically high or low, though high is more common. When your cortisol levels are off, they can trigger autoimmune disorders along with food and chemical intolerances.

They can also disrupt reproductive hormones and thyroid hormone activity. Furthermore, chronically high cortisol induces intestinal permeability (leaky gut), which causes more food intolerances, digestive problems, and intestinal inflammation. Controlling your cortisol is key in repairing the intestinal lining to help improve digestion.

Cortisol imbalances are brought on by chronic stress. The first step is to find the source of the chronic stress. It may be sleep deprivation, a bad relationship, a toxic work environment, or something else. Stress manifests in a lot of ways, and you can't ignore it. It's sure to come out in some way, large or subtle, that can be detrimental to your health, cause inflammation, and create further issues down the road.

If stress is unavoidable, you can mitigate the stress in several small ways: ensure you're getting enough sleep, make time to exercise, meditate, go on walks, and/or socialize and spend time with friends and family. Finding what helps alleviate your own stress is just as important as figuring out the source of it.

ESTROGEN

Estrogen is responsible for the regulation and development of a woman's reproductive system. When estrogen levels are off—whether estrogen is too high, too low, or, worst of all, constantly fluctuating as it does during perimenopause—women may experience inflammatory issues and other challenges. Symptoms of hormonal imbalances in women include irregular cycles, PMS, infertility, PCOS, and a difficult time transitioning into menopause. A lot of women who were healthy for most of their lives may nosedive when going through menopause as these inflammatory pathways are triggered and become really hard to regulate.

Calming your inflammation helps regulate estrogen, which will make the transition to menopause easier.

INSULIN

Insulin is a hormone that helps regulate blood sugar by escorting glucose into cells to be used for energy. Many of our chronic inflammation and autoimmune patients have chronically high insulin, which is a precursor to diabetes. High insulin also creates an inflammatory state in the body and brain.

Insulin resistance is a big issue for inflammation. Aside from high blood sugar, the most common signs of insulin resistance are excess belly fat, feeling sleepy after meals, and poor sleep. The steps you take to dampen inflammation will be the same ones you use to reverse insulin resistance and lower blood sugar, which I talk about in part two of this book.

ENVIRONMENTAL TOXINS & HOW TO BUFFER THEM

We live in a sea of thousands of synthetic and toxic environmental chemicals. They exist in the air we breathe, the water we drink, and the soil in which we grow our food (yes, even organic ones). There are toxins in body products, makeup, and hair products, as well as furniture, flooring, and building materials that off-gas toxins. Although we may not absorb toxins in amounts great enough to immediately poison and kill us, they accumulate in our bodies, adding to our overall body burden. Multiple studies show people carry toxins in their bodies, and they have been found in breast milk and even in fetal placenta cords.

The Inflammatory Reset gives you an action plan to support your body as a toxin biotransformation machine, but minimizing your exposure to toxins is a vital part of managing inflammation and autoimmunity. For instance, even if you eat all the right foods and live an anti-inflammatory lifestyle but drink hot drinks through plastic lids or microwave your meals in plastic, you could unwittingly be provoking your inflammation through toxic exposure.

In this chapter, Karalynne Call—a certified nutritionist and mental health advocate of the popular Instagram page *@just.ingredients* and its podcast—discusses seven kinds of **endocrine disruptors**. Endocrine disruptors are chemicals that disrupt how our hormones function by mimicking the structure of natural hormones, confusing the body, or altering how hormones function. As some of the most common forms of toxins we encounter in our everyday lives, they are strongly linked to inflammation. It's important to learn how they affect our health and how to minimize exposure.

BPA & BPS

Bisphenol A (BPA) and bisphenol S (BPS) are chemical cousins that are commonly found in food- and beverage-can linings, other food-packaging materials, certain polycarbonate plastic bottles, and cash register

ENVIRONMENTAL TOXINS & HOW TO BUFFER THEM

receipts. It is also a residue found in our tap water. BPS was the replacement chemical for BPA in products that are BPA-free, but it is more potent in terms of hazard.

Unfortunately, this plastic acts as a synthetic hormone and can trick the body into thinking it's the real thing—and the results aren't pretty. Both BPA and BPS disrupt the endocrine system and create an inflammatory response. BPA has been linked to breast and other cancers, reproductive problems, obesity, early puberty, and heart disease.

They are ubiquitous, even in our bodies. According to government tests, 93% of Americans have BPA in their bodies, and a separate study in 2015–2016 found 97% of participants had BPA in their urine samples. Compared to bodies that have none, bodies with BPA in urine have a 21% increase in inflammatory markers. BPA raises inflammation by increasing the production of cytokines (inflammatory immune cells).

HOW TO AVOID BPA & BPS

- Use glass food storage instead of plastic (yes, no more Tupperware).
- Never heat anything in plastic or cans.
- Use a water filter.
- Say no to receipts, since thermal paper is often coated with BPS or BPA.
- Avoid plastics marked with "PC" (for polycarbonate) or recycling label #7. Not all of these plastics contain BPA, but many do.
- Use fresh, frozen, or dried food instead of canned food.
- Check whether a food or beverage package contains BPA using the Environmental Working Group's (EWG) BPA product list. You can find alternatives in EWG's Food Scores.
- Quit drinking out of plastic water bottles and use stainless steel or glass.
- Avoid plastic dishware and use ceramic, bamboo, stainless steel, or glass.
- Avoid plastic cooking utensils and use stainless steel or bamboo.

- Use silicone storage bags instead of plastic.
- Use glass baby bottles instead of plastic.
- Use wooden toys instead of plastic.

DIOXINS

Dioxins are a group of chemical compounds that form, most often, from incomplete burning of household and industrial waste. They also can be produced during bleaching of paper pulp and the manufacture of certain chlorinated chemicals like polychlorinated biphenyls (PCBs), chlorinated phenols, chlorinated benzene, and certain pesticides. Exhaust from vehicles, forest fires, and burning wood also release dioxins into the air.

Dioxins live long, with a half-life of seven to eleven years. They build up in the body and in the food chain, meaning the higher an animal is in the food chain, the higher the concentration of dioxins. At the top of most food chains are humans.

Dioxins are well studied, and research shows that they are some of the most proinflammatory toxins in the environment, commonly inducing chronic inflammation in the body. This immune activation directly influences male and female reproductive systems, lowering sperm quality and count in males and promoting endometriosis in females. In terms of reproduction, damage can start in utero when the fetus is exposed to even low levels of dioxins, which can disrupt hormone signaling and reproductive development.

HOW TO AVOID DIOXINS

- Eat fewer animal-based products. One study shows those who eat a plant-based diet have the least amount of dioxin exposure.
- Eat more veggies. Phytonutrients from a heavy plant-based diet will help arm the body against dioxin exposure.
- Eat less farmed fish and buy wild fish whenever possible.
- Eat organic veggies and fruit, especially those listed on EWG's annual "The Dirty Dozen" list.
- Use organic cotton and paper-based products wherever possible.

- Avoid using bleached tampons, sanitary pads, or toilet paper. Use unbleached paper towels, parchment paper, coffee filters, and other products.

- Take your shoes off before entering homes, wash your clothes if you've been out in the garden, and wash veggies and fruits picked from the garden. Do not use Roundup and other toxic pesticides.

- Use an air filter in your home.

PARABENS

Parabens—synthetic preservatives that extend shelf life and hinder the growth of bacteria—are used in a variety of products, including cosmetics, pharmaceuticals, and food. They reach the bloodstream through ingestion or through permeation of the skin when applied topically and can trigger inflammation, disrupt hormone balance, impact fertility and reproductive organs, and affect birth outcomes.

Parabens are also endocrine disruptors through their hormone-mimicking properties and have been found in breast cancer cells, suggesting they mimic estrogen once in the bloodstream. One study detected traces of five parabens in the breast tumors of 19 out of 20 women.

The most common parabens include methyl-, ethyl-, propyl-, isopropyl-, butyl-, and isobutylparaben. These endocrine disruptors are often found in the following personal care products:

- Products with a leave-on, rinse-off nature, especially those with a high water content, such as shampoos and conditioners.

- Condoms and lubricants (the permeable and sensitive skin of the vagina is likely to absorb parabens in this way).

- Moisturizers, face and skin cleaners, sunscreens, deodorants, shaving gels, toothpastes, makeup, and many other body products.

Researchers have also found measurable amounts of parabens in some 90% of typical grocery items—such as beers, sauces, desserts, soft drinks, jams, pickles, frozen dairy products, processed vegetables, and flavoring

THE INFLAMMATORY RESET

syrups—which is why those who steer clear of potentially harmful personal care products still carry parabens around in their bloodstreams.

HOW TO AVOID PARABENS

- *Always* read the ingredients on your cosmetics and personal care products.
- Learn to identify the six most common parabens (methyl-, ethyl-, propyl-, isopropyl-, butyl- and isobutylparaben). Look for products that have certified "paraben-free" labels.
- Avoid purchasing common name brands that use parabens for their formulas, such as Bath & Body Works, CeraVe, Neutrogena, Maybelline, Cover Girl, Arm & Hammer, Degree, Aveeno, Ponds, and Cetaphil.
- Choose a nontoxic lubricant such as Sustain Natural or Coconu.
- User dryer balls instead of dryer sheets.
- Familiarize yourself with products that aren't shelf-stable forever—that's okay! That's how you know it's fresh and not filled with synthetic preservatives.
- Shop local and buy in small batches. Avoid boxed, canned, and packaged foods.
- Make jams, sauces, syrups, etc. *from home.*
- Use resources like EWG to cross-check products.

PHTHALATES

Known as "the everywhere chemical," phthalates are a group of chemicals that make plastics flexible and hard to break. They are easily concealed because of their sightless, odorless composition, and are often listed in the ingredients as just "fragrance." These are the most commonly used phthalates:

- Diethyl phthalate (DEP)
- Di-n-butyl phthalate (DBP)
- Diisobutyl phthalate (DIBP)

- Dimethyl phthalate (DMP)
- Diisohexyl phthalate (DIHP)
- Di-n-hexyl phthalate (DnHP)
- Di-n-octyl phthalate (DnOP)

Phthalates are released into the environment during production, through usage, and with disposal. They migrate easily and are readily absorbed through the skin. Exposure to phthalates has been found to induce inflammation and cause an inflammatory response in the endocrine system. Similar to parabens, they are major endocrine disruptors, impacting the reproductive system and hormones in women, men, and children. Phthalates are linked with altered development of genitals, low sperm count, and poor sperm quality. Studies suggest that high levels of phthalates can lead to premature delivery in pregnant women. Phthalates also cross through the placenta. You can find them in a lot of places too:

- Commonly used plastics, including plastic food storage containers, plastic dishware, PVC piping, air plug-ins, car air fresheners, grocery bags, garbage bags, shower curtains, toys, inflatable mattresses, three-ring binders, diaper mats, paints and primers, crafts, outdoor hoses, party favors, and plastic jewelry.
- Pharmaceuticals.
- Household cosmetics, usually listed as "fragrance" in shampoo, conditioner, and hairsprays. Also in nail polish, deodorant, perfume, and makeup.
- Food packaging.
- Water and beverage bottles.
- Infant formula.

HOW TO AVOID PHTHALATES

- Read all ingredient labels on food packaging, cleaning supplies, soaps, detergents, and cosmetics. Look for phthalates disguised as "fragrance" or "parfum."

THE INFLAMMATORY RESET

- Avoid *all* synthetic fragrances in everything you use. Stop using plug-ins and air fresheners. Switch out perfumes and colognes for products made with natural fragrances, such as Beauty By Earth.
- Avoid plastic containers labeled with a "3" within the recycling arrows, as well as the letters "V" and "PVC." In choosing plastic products, look for numbers 1, 2, 4, and 5 within the arrows.
- Make food from home as much as possible. Processed foods are exposed to a significant amount of phthalates.

PFAS (PERFLUOROALKYL & POLYFLUOROALKYL SUBSTANCES)

Per- and polyfluoroalkyl substances (PFAS) are a group of chemicals that include PFOA, PFOS, GenX, and many others. They don't break down easily and are very persistent in both the environment and the human body, where they accumulate. In fact, research shows that 99% of Americans have PFAS in their bodies.

Exposure to PFAS has been linked to decreased sperm quality, low birth weight, kidney disease, thyroid disease, and high cholesterol, among other health issues. These chemicals cause stress in the body, which can cause inflammation.

Often referred to as the "forever chemicals" because they don't break down under typical circumstances, PFAS have made their way into soil and, in some places, our drinking water. In short, they are all around us. One of the most recognizable sources of PFAS is Teflon nonstick cookware. They're also in food wrappers, packaged foods, tents, carpets, umbrellas, and polishes and cleaning products. Most lakes, rivers, reservoirs, landfills, and treatment plants also have huge amounts of PFA residues.

HOW TO AVOID PFAS

- Avoid Teflon or nonstick cookware. If you choose to continue using nonstick cookware, be careful not to let it heat above 450°F. Do not leave nonstick cookware unattended on the stove or use it in hot ovens or on grills. Use cast-iron, 100% ceramic, or high-quality stainless-steel cookware.

- Avoid stain-resistant treatments and choose furniture and carpets that aren't marketed as "stain-resistant." Do not apply finishing treatments such as Stainmaster to these or other items.

- Avoid greasy or oily packaged and fast foods—the packaging often contains grease-repellent coatings that contain PFAS. Examples include microwave popcorn bags and fast-food wrappers.

- Avoid personal care products made with Teflon or containing ingredients that include the words "fluoro" or "perfluoro." PFAS can be found in dental floss and a variety of cosmetics, including nail polish, facial moisturizers, and eye makeup.

GLYPHOSATE

Glyphosate is the main active ingredient in Roundup, the most widely used herbicide in the United States. Roundup is used on wheat, corn, soybean, oat, and other crops before harvesting. Glyphosate kills the crop, drying it out uniformly so that it can be harvested earlier and more easily. Strangely, glyphosate was patented as an antibiotic. It's unfortunately very effective against some of the most beneficial gut flora our bodies need.

Glyphosate is found in so many products today that most of us carry a significant amount in our bodies, contributing to stress and chronic inflammation. Studies suggest even relatively low levels of glyphosate may be endocrine disruptors with the ability to potentially reduce testosterone levels, impair sperm quality, or cause disturbances in reproductive development. In one study, the offspring of rats exposed to glyphosate had altered gut microbiota in early development. Some major sources include meats and animal products, produce, grains, corn, almonds, commercially produced dairy milks, soy, hummus, beans, and lentils.

HOW TO AVOID GLYPHOSATE

- Buy organic veggies and fruit whenever you can. If you can, buy from local organic farmers to ensure you know the source and how fresh it is.

THE INFLAMMATORY RESET

- Buy organic grains. This includes organic processed grains such as breads, crackers, tortillas, cereals, pasta, rice, chips, etc.
- Opt for 100% grass-fed and grass-finished meats, if possible.
- Buy organic nuts and organic nut-based products such as almond milk, almond flour, and almond butter.
- Avoid using Roundup or other toxic pesticides and insecticides on your property. There are much cleaner and healthier options.

FLAME RETARDANTS

Flame retardants are used on many products today, including our furniture. Polybrominated diphenyl ethers (PBDEs) and Tetrabromobisphenol A (TBBPA) make up the majority of flame retardants. These powerful and toxic agents are significant endocrine and thyroid disruptors that impact immune and reproductive function, raise the risk of cancer, and affect fetal and child development and neurologic functions.

One of the biggest dangers of some flame retardants is that they bioaccumulate in humans, promoting chronic inflammation and long-term health problems. Flame retardants are most commonly found in carpets, fabric blinds, mattresses, furniture foam, textiles, car seats (infant and toddler), and gym foam blocks.

They are so widespread that they've also made their way into some of our food sources. The top four food sources include meat, fish, dairy, and eggs.

HOW TO AVOID FLAME RETARDANTS

- Avoid things that use the term "flame retardant" and look for "flame retardant-free."
- When looking to purchase furniture, car seats, mattresses, baby products, or other items, search the internet to see if they are treated with flame retardants.
- Look for brands that have banned flame retardants completely from their inventory.

COVID & INFLAMMATION

In the years following the Covid-19 pandemic, some people still suffer with chronic symptoms from Covid and are called Covid long-haulers. For anyone already dealing with inflammation, this additional response further compounds the stress on the body. The good news is that the same set of approaches outlined in this book can reset and reduce that inflammation, balancing immune health by addressing the whole health of the body.

Many people think of Covid as being similar to the flu or a cold, but it has unique symptoms and consequences. The science is fascinating, but to make it brief: Covid has amino acid sequences that are identical to those in some body tissues. This means that when the immune system attacks the virus, it can also mistakenly attack the identical amino acid sequences in your body tissue, creating an autoimmune reaction that persists long after you've recovered from Covid.

People who experience this autoimmune response initially see a rise in blood pressure, inflammation, and tissue damage throughout the body, along with potential damage to the lining of the blood vessels. Researchers have found that Covid damages endothelial tissue, affecting the lungs, kidney, heart, small intestines, pancreas, brain, and so forth. Damage to these tissues can create long-term effects and worsen pre-existing health conditions.

What's more, in many people, Covid also produces a cytokine storm. Inflammatory cytokines fight infections; however, Covid patients produce an exaggerated inflammatory response and an overabundance of cytokines. Some people who were sick months or even years ago show that they are still very inflamed on blood tests. The increased inflammation and cytokine storms cause the brain to become inflamed, which impairs brain function and speeds up the degeneration of brain tissue, going beyond the duration of your basic Covid infection.

THE INFLAMMATORY RESET

If you've had unusual and chronic symptoms post-Covid, it's important to validate your experience, even if the people in your life fail to do so, and listen to trusted medical professionals. There's a lot of information and opinions out there, not all with your health in mind.

If you see markers for elevated inflammation on a blood test, you can use simple diet, lifestyle, and nutrition strategies to calm down the inflammation. While there are many causes of inflammation and ways you can experience it, the solutions are all the same. For those suffering with Covid long-hauler symptoms, the Inflammatory Reset can potentially get you back on your feet.

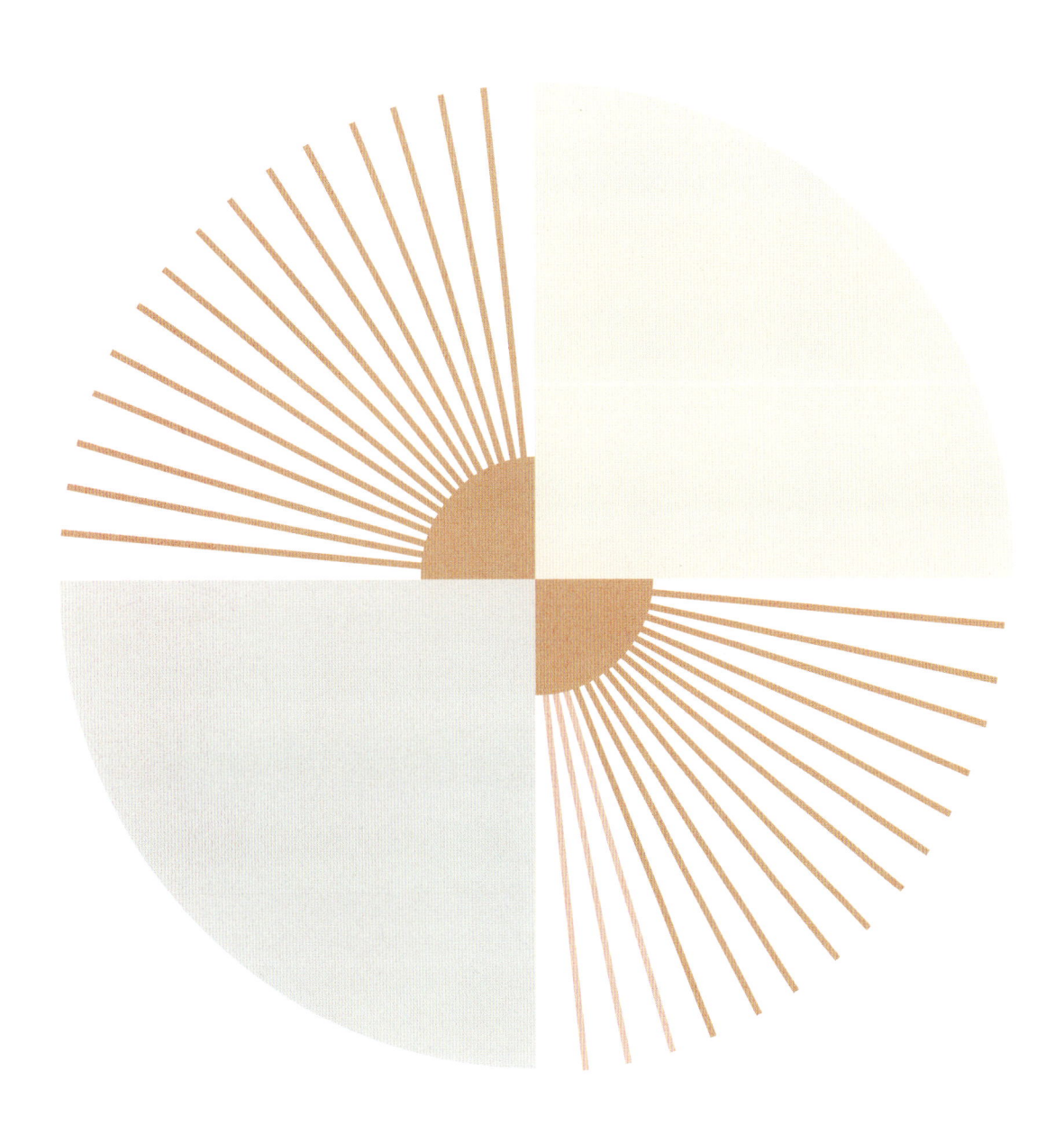

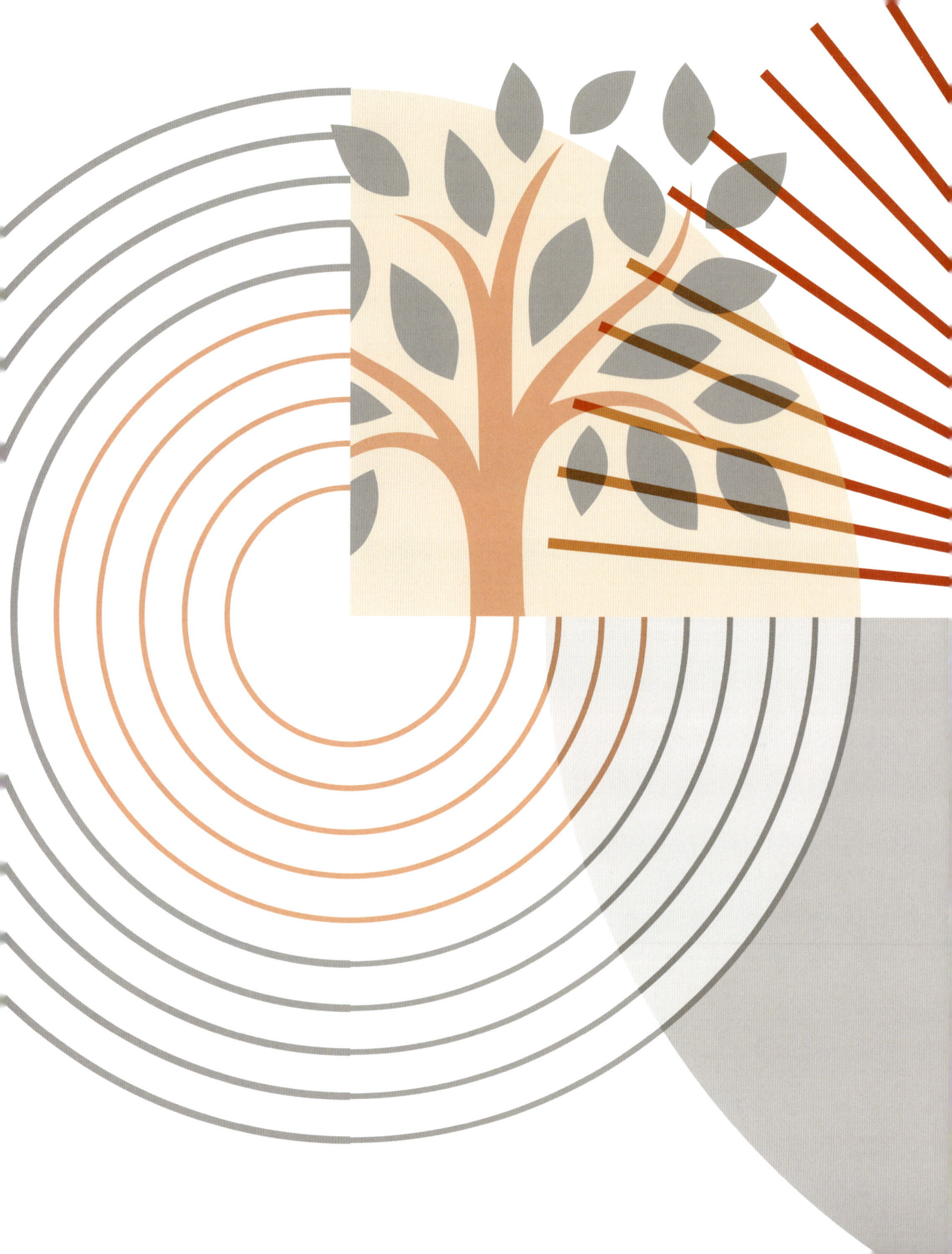

PART TWO

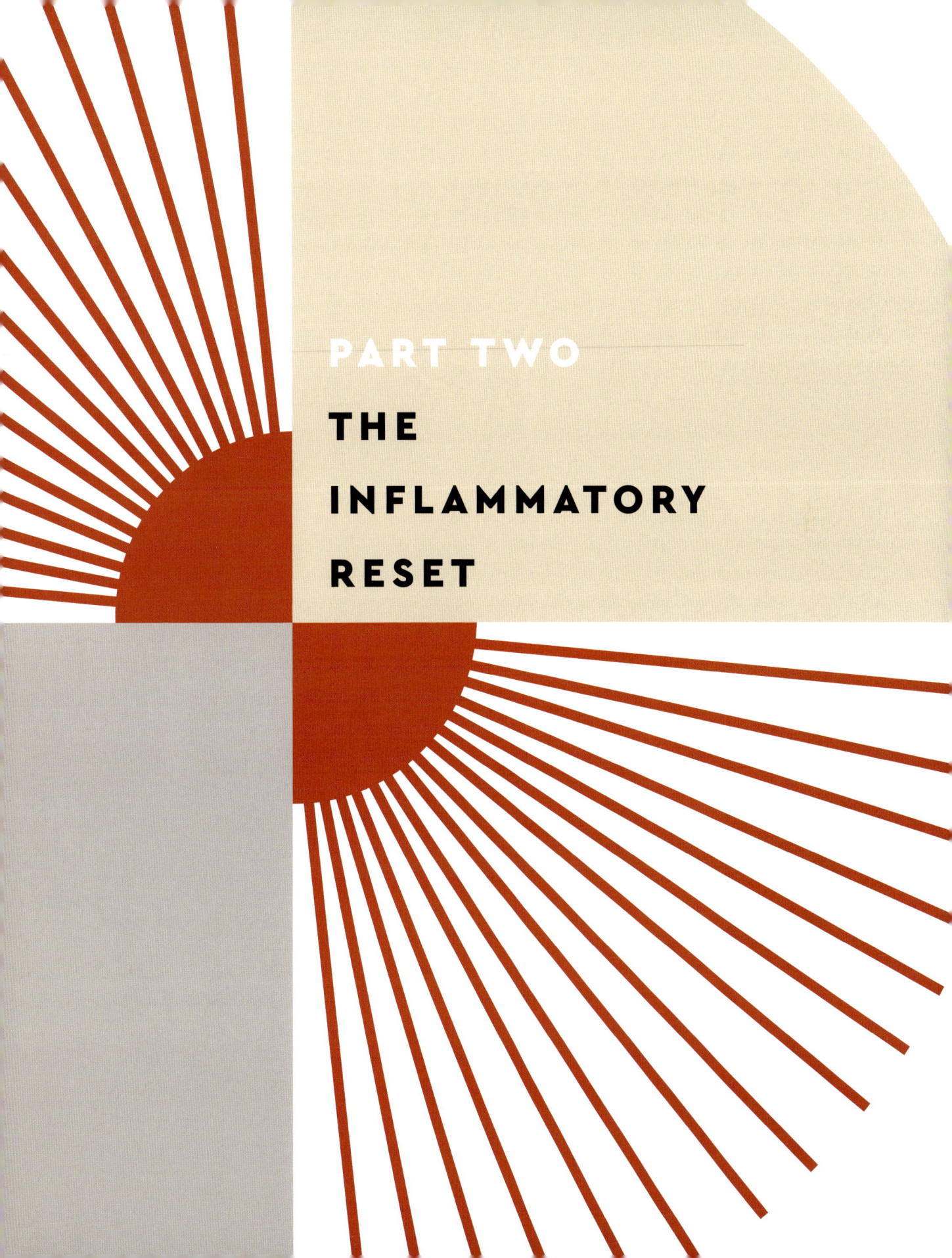

THE INFLAMMATORY RESET

THE INFLAMMATORY RESET

The Inflammatory Reset is a program that I've been working on for a while. For over 10 years, my goal has been to give you the tools to maintain your own health, which will minimize unnecessary doctor visits for you. It's probably not the best business model for me, but I hope you can take these practices and apply them to your life.

I've designed the Inflammatory Reset to be a 30-day program in which you learn to change your exercise routine, behaviors, and diet, all with the intention of learning how your individual body experiences inflammation and how to reduce it.

Resetting your inflammation is a multipronged approach, requiring effort in every area; you can't just do one and expect results. Though it's designed as a 30-day program, some people stick it out longer and implement a majority of the changes into their lives long-term.

In sticking to the Inflammatory Reset and practicing these specific exercises for a month, you will see significant decreases in the inflammation in your body. It can be hard to stick to a strict regimen, but I know you can do it. Each passing day gets easier as you wean your body off the inflammatory foods it craves and incorporate lifestyle changes and exercises to become healthier.

ACTIVITIES & EXERCISES TO REDUCE INFLAMMATION

The Inflammatory Reset requires more than changes to your diet; lifestyle choices are just as important. In my research and clinic practices, we do a range of exercises and activities with our patients to help reduce inflammation. Modern technology has gifted us with amazing ways to treat inflammation, along with classic staples like daily exercise that are great for your health and inflammation simultaneously.

A LIFESTYLE TO REDUCE INFLAMMATION

Reducing inflammation begins with examining your everyday routines and actions. No dietary change or activity can really function or fulfill its potential without the foundation of a healthy and balanced anti-inflammatory lifestyle. There are several major areas to prioritize:

- Getting enough sleep. Sleep deprivation not only makes you tired, it also increases stress, worsens brain function, and spikes inflammation. The brain uses sleep for growth and repair. Sleep is foundational to good immune function, good brain health, and dampening inflammation.

- Managing and understanding trauma. As I mentioned, trauma can cause inflammation in recurring and unknown ways. Finding the source can be difficult, and I highly recommend working with a therapist to help discover and alleviate these sources of inflammation.

- Managing stress. Stress manifests in various ways. It's important to locate the cause of it in order to reduce your inflammation. Avoiding toxic situations (including relationships and people) and controlling your work-life balance are important steps to take in your anti-inflammatory journey.

THE INFLAMMATORY RESET

- Keeping a regular eating and sleeping schedule. When you eat and sleep at inconsistent hours, your body reacts in a defensive and inflammatory way. With a consistent eating and sleeping routine, your body naturally mitigates and manages inflammation.

- Removing the inflammatory home and body products from your household. As Karalynne discussed earlier, removing inflammatory products and seeking better, often more natural alternatives helps reduce your inflammation in subtle yet significant ways.

These basic steps form the groundwork to reduce your inflammation. When you change your routine for the better, your chances of making the Inflammatory Reset successful improve drastically.

EXERCISE

Daily exercise may initially seem like a bad idea when you feel run down, in pain, or fatigued from chronic inflammation. However, studies show daily physical activity helps manage symptoms from inflammation compared to not exercising at all. This even extends to patients who may stop exercising due to pain, such as those with rheumatoid arthritis. No matter how small the effort, any regular physical activity is better than none.

Additionally, people who engage in regular physical activity report less depression, better self-esteem, and increased happiness. These benefits alone support a positive mindset, which is anti-inflammatory compared to a negative one.

High-intensity interval training (HIIT), in particular, dilates blood vessels, lowers inflammation, and improves blood flow to the brain. HIIT involves reaching your maximum heart rate with a short but vigorous burst of exercise, resting, and repeating. You push yourself until you're out of breath at 70%–90% of maximum heart rate, recover at 60%–65% of maximum heart rate, and then do it again about five to seven times in a row. (There are a couple of ways to determine your maximum heart rate, but a quick rule of thumb is subtracting your age from 220.) This can be done on a spin bike, running, walking up a hill, doing calisthenics, or whatever works for you. Even just a few minutes of high-intensity exercise daily can improve blood flow in the

ACTIVITIES & EXERCISES TO REDUCE INFLAMMATION

brain. My autoimmune patients see the best results when they do at least 15 minutes of HIIT first thing in the morning every day.

If someone has a severe autoimmune disease or a severe inflammatory condition, exercise initially may make things worse because it increases exercise-induced cytokines, which create an inflammatory response and can exacerbate symptoms. With our patients, we have to be cautious with the intensity and length of exercise. Once the inflammation has calmed down, bodily functions are back to normal, and the patient's body has become used to the exercise, we can then increase the intensity and duration of exercise without excess flare-ups.

While exercise is vital, overexercising increases inflammation and weakens the immune system, so don't overdo it. Some people can walk outside for 10 minutes first thing in the morning. Others can do more. What's important is that you listen to your body and understand your limits. Once the inflammation and autoimmune responses calm down, you can extend duration and increase intensity cautiously and slowly.

MEDITATION

Meditation and other mindfulness practices can improve your emotional well-being and the health of your subconscious "operating system." Other mindfulness practices include deep breathing exercises, yoga, and tai chi. Even 10 minutes a day is shown to increase concentration and overall calmness. There are apps like Headspace, Calm, and many more to help you meditate and boost your mental health.

Many people feel that it's hard to find time or feel like they're doing it well. I won't tell you I nailed mindfulness and meditation on my first try, but I did feel better after some practice. I like to think that one minute is better than nothing. Start small and be consistent—you don't have to do a whole half hour in silence. Meditation can be medicine. It's about having some time for yourself, letting that nervous system calm down, and helping to reduce that inflammation.

THE INFLAMMATORY RESET

STIMULATING THE VAGUS NERVE

The **vagus nerve** is a large nerve that runs between the brain and the organs of the body. Stimulating the vagus nerve can improve function of the organs and metabolic systems, such as digestive health, as well as activate the brain to improve brain health and reduce brain inflammation. Studies also show that stimulating the vagus nerve helps dampen overall inflammation and symptoms of autoimmune disorders.

It can also activate the parasympathetic nervous system—the rest-and-digest system—which improves gut health and enhances focus and relaxation. Because of these many benefits, I am a huge fan of doing exercises that can activate the vagus-nerve highway running through your body. These are some of the exercises I recommend:

- Gargle aggressively. Gargle water as intensely as possible for three minutes, three times a day.

- Sing loudly. If you are alone at home or in the car, spend some time singing as loudly as you can.

- Make yourself gag. Using a tongue depressor, gently press on the back of your tongue to make yourself gag, without poking the back of your throat. Do this three times a day during your reset.

- Practice deep breathing exercises. Deep breathing helps stimulate the vagus nerve, improves lung capacity, and oxygenates the body. During the Inflammatory Reset, do this three times a day for five minutes at a time, breathe as deeply as you can through your nose and exhale out your mouth. The goal is to minimize how many breaths you take per minute. Count your breaths and see if you can work toward cutting them in half.

ICE BATHS & COLD SHOWERS

Many people with inflammation struggle with mornings due to sluggish brain function, but this is the time of day you should feel most alert. Taking an ice bath or cold shower first thing in the morning will help stimulate the cortisol awakening response (CAR) and adrenal function to set the day off right. You may have

ACTIVITIES & EXERCISES TO REDUCE INFLAMMATION

reservations about this idea, but even two to three minutes in an ice bath in the morning or just one minute in a cold shower with deep breathing can stimulate an anti-inflammatory cholinergic pathway that will dampen inflammation.

For this to work, shower on the coldest setting for at least one minute. If you plan to take a hot shower as well, you can switch to cold after your hot shower, but not before. If you have a bathtub, fill it with ice and submerge yourself. Start with 30 seconds and work yourself up from there.

I also suggest doing breathing exercises along with the cold-water therapy—this will help you tolerate the temperature in the beginning. Keep it simple by focusing on long, slow breaths. Use the experience to lengthen and deepen your breathing exercises, eventually working toward as few breaths as possible. All of this will improve vagus nerve function, oxygenate your body better, and improve your lung capacity.

You will also find the cold showers and ice baths give you a sense of accomplishment, which boosts dopamine that in turn boosts mood, motivation, and energy. Although they sound horrible, most people come around to morning cold showers or ice baths for how much better it makes them feel.

INFRARED SAUNA

One of the most powerful tools for pain relief, detoxification, inflammation, and heart health is a far-infrared sauna. Conventional hot rock and steam saunas simply heat the air, while far-infrared light saunas penetrate tissue. This releases stored toxins, improves metabolism, and oxygenates the body.

Seek out "far-infrared saunas" when looking for them in your area and use these two to four times a week, starting with 10–15 minute sessions and slowly working your way up to 30–40 minutes.

ALPHA-STIM TRAINING

Your brain naturally has electrical currents. You can stimulate and modulate specific groups of nerve cells with the Alpha-Stim cranial electrotherapy stimulation (CES) device, which delivers a natural level of microcurrent via small clips worn on your earlobes.

The microcurrent is very tiny and completely safe and is effective for anxiety relief, mood normalization, and better sleep in both quality and duration.

Not only does the Alpha-Stim improve brain function, it also has been shown to relieve post-traumatic stress and acute and chronic pain. Treatments often take only 20 minutes and you can use Alpha-Stim in the privacy of your own home or carry it with you. I recommend doing it daily, although you can wear it for as long as you want if you need additional support. You can order one online at alpha-stim.com.

HYPERBARIC OXYGEN THERAPY

Hyperbaric oxygen therapy (HBOT) involves lying comfortably in a pressurized oxygen-rich environment. This increased pressure in oxygen-rich air allows the oxygen to dissolve and saturate your blood plasma, exponentially increasing the delivery of oxygen throughout your body and allowing it to reach inflamed tissues and infuse the body's cells for improved function. The chronically inflamed and autoimmune patients we see in our clinics have achieved great results using HBOT for treatment.

HBOT treatments are expensive and intensive, but if your condition is advanced, you may find it worth the investment. Typically, people go in five days a week for 10 to 40 sessions total.

RESETTING YOUR DIET

Changing up your diet may not be easy, but it is one of the most effective ways to change the course of your life. In managing inflammation, most of our patients end up eating healthier as a whole, which doubles down on cutting out the inflammatory foods.

We encourage people in our clinics to start reading nutrition labels and to pay particular attention to the list of ingredients. Many foods that are marketed to be "healthy," "all-natural," "organic," "fat-free," or "sugar-free" have numerous ingredients that you will need to avoid while on the Inflammatory Reset diet and should just avoid altogether.

We've put together a list of foods for you to eliminate and a list of those to add to your diet for the next 30 days. One of the more common gripes we hear is that the list of foods to avoid cuts out gluten, dairy, pork, and beef. If you're asking yourself what you are supposed to eat, you're probably stuck in an inflammatory food trap. I know those are big asks to go without, but there are still many foods you can eat, and many healthier options you should add to your diet. We want to make the Inflammatory Reset as accessible as possible for you, and that's why we've included a whole cookbook.

THE INFLAMMATORY RESET

FOODS TO AVOID

Not everyone reacts to these, as everyone is unique with food intolerances, but this is a good place to start and reset before you decide to reintroduce foods. If you have severe inflammation or autoimmune diseases, we recommend avoiding all nuts, seeds, beans, nightshades, peas, and all legumes for the first two weeks in addition to the foods listed here.

- Any food you are allergic to
- Dairy, including milk, cheese, yogurt, butter, margarine, and shortening
- Eggs
- Gluten: wheat, oats, rye, and barley, typically found in breads, pasta, and cereals
- Tomatoes, tomato sauces, and anything containing tomatoes
- Dehydrated fruit
- Rice, corn, potatoes (white, red, yellow)
- Alcohol
- Coffee, black tea, and soda, both caffeinated and caffeine-free
- Fruit juices
- Iodized (table) salt
- Sugar, along with natural and artificial sweeteners, including agave
- Soy or products containing soy, including soy milk and tofu
- Peanuts, including peanut butter and peanut oil
- Beef, pork, shellfish, cold cuts, bacon, hot dogs, canned meat, and sausage

RESETTING YOUR DIET

FOODS TO EAT

You may feel a little overwhelmed seeing all the foods you can no longer eat in the previous section, but there are many great foods you can have in your Inflammatory Reset. I encourage you to try a variety of things to see what you enjoy.

- Chicken, turkey, and lamb in moderate amounts
- Fish (except shellfish)
- Quinoa and buckwheat (without wheat or gluten additives)
- Sweet potatoes in moderate amounts
- Peas (split, fresh, and snap)
- Beans, including navy, white, kidney, garbanzo, black, etc.
- Raw cashews, almonds, macadamia nuts, sunflower seeds, pecans, and walnuts
- Fresh fruits and vegetables
- Herbal teas and decaffeinated green teas
- Unsweetened coconut milk, almond milk, and cashew milk
- Olive oil, coconut oil, avocado oil, and flaxseed oil in moderate amounts
- Sea salt and spices (individual spices are less likely to have intolerable additives than spice blends)

REINTRODUCING ELIMINATED FOODS

After following an anti-inflammatory diet and seeing an improvement in your symptoms and health, you may decide to reintroduce some foods. It's crucial to monitor your symptoms when reintroducing foods. Reactions vary from person to person when having an immune response to food: the problematic food could affect your brain function, energy levels, skin, and so on.

Be aware of anything that seems to exacerbate symptoms, no matter how trivial. The moment your body reacts negatively to a food you reintroduced, immediately stop eating it. Return to your previous diet until you feel well. If you'd like to reintroduce another food, wait until you are at your "baseline," or back to feeling how you felt at the end of your 30-day anti-inflammatory diet, before you began reintroducing foods.

Reintroduce one food at a time so you don't confuse any reactions. Additionally, like individual symptoms, you need to understand what your particular flare-ups feel like. Again, everyone's reactions are unique, and the sooner you recognize yours, the sooner you can figure out what foods work best for you.

SUPPLEMENTS & INFLAMMATION

Supplements, as the name suggests, are add-ons to your diet and regimen of exercise; to be clear, *no amount of supplements can outrun a poor diet*. That being said, I recommend my patients start out on the following supplements to augment the Inflammatory Reset.

Supplement	Use(s)	Dosage	Notes
Turmeric	Dampens inflammation and improves integrity of the intestinal and blood-brain barriers.	How much you take depends on how bad inflammation is, so take enough to feel an effect. My favorite products are Turmeric Complex by Just Ingredients, which contains organic turmeric, organic resveratrol, and boswellia, or TurmeraSorb XL by PalmaVita Therapeutics.	Should contain black pepper to enhance bioavailability and absorption. Research shows black pepper can improve the absorption of turmeric by up to 2000%.
Resveratrol	Dampens inflammation.	Again, how much you take depends on how bad inflammation is, so take enough to feel an effect. My favorite products are Turmeric Complex by Just Ingredients, which contains organic turmeric, organic resveratrol, and boswellia, or ResveraSorb XL by PalmaVita Therapeutics.	Should contain black pepper to enhance bioavailability and absorption. Research shows black pepper can improve the absorption of resveratrol by up to 154% and boswellia by up to 20 times more.
Vitamin D	Supplements your vitamin D levels, which inflammation inhibits.	Use the cholecalciferol D3 form. I recommend D3 + K2 by Just Ingredients or Bioavaili-D by PalmaVita Therapeutics.	

THE INFLAMMATORY RESET

Supplement	Use(s)	Dosage	Notes
Glutathione	Protects brain and body cells from inflammatory damage. As an antioxidant, it protects your cells against free radicals. It also protects you from the toxins in our environment, stresses, and the difficulties associated with aging.	I recommend Fortizome 3X from PalmaVita Therapeutics. How much you need depends on the degree of your inflammation, but we have our patients take 5–10 ml three times a day. You can also boost your body's ability to make glutathione by taking 600 to 900 mg of n-acetyl-cysteine twice a day. You can also undergo glutathione IV therapy.	People over age 50 should be taking this daily.

A WORD ON VITAMIN D

Vitamin D is a negative acute phase reactant, which is a very technical way of saying that under inflammation, vitamin D decreases. This is not a good thing. Vitamin D helps increase the amount of regulatory T cells (Tregs) that, as their name implies, regulate T cell proliferation.

On the other hand, T cells are our immune champions. When your body is confronted with dangerous bacteria or viruses, T cells flourish to combat the infection in an autoimmune response. At this time, it would be bad to take vitamin D, because your body needs all those T cells, and you don't want to dampen the count.

However, when someone has chronic inflammation, vitamin D is chronically low. Taking additional vitamin D helps foster more regulatory T cells, suppress T cell increases, and mitigate autoimmune responses.

SUPPLEMENTS & INFLAMMATION

A WORD ON CBD & CANNABIS

If you google "CBD" or "cannabis," you'll be overwhelmed with articles touting the medicinal benefits of cannabidiol (CBD) and cannabis for all kinds of health disorders. While these compounds have indeed shown great benefits, people with inflammation and autoimmunity should be careful as they can cause inflammation and flare-ups in some.

CBD and cannabis can potentially help with conditions such as epilepsy, arthritis, autoimmunity, Parkinson's, anxiety, depression, mood, inflammation, and so much more. Numerous studies are being conducted to discover what they can help and alleviate. However, there are three main reasons why CBD or cannabis can have a negative effect in some people:

1. Some people may have an allergic reaction or intolerance to the Cannabaceae family of flowering plants.
2. Some marijuana strains stimulate inflammatory T cells, exacerbating an autoimmune response.
3. Because the products aren't farmed organically, people can react to pesticides and poor farming techniques.

Of the more than 1,000 strains of cannabis and CBD, some strains activate an immune response that can worsen autoimmunity. Typically, the best strains for pain and inflammation are those that have higher amounts of CBD to THC. CBD is the compound best known for fighting pain and inflammation.

I'm not saying not to use CBD. In fact, I have become a regular user of and advocate for CBD for back pain after fracturing my back and becoming partially paralyzed for a few days. Just be conscious of the strains you're using and the reactions your body has to each one.

SAMPLE PROTOCOL

We've thrown a lot of information at you thus far regarding what to do, what to eat, and what to take to reduce your inflammation. It's a lot to take in, so I've created something of a sample protocol for you to follow or use as a base for your own plan, if you'd like.

Everyone's anti-inflammatory journey is unique, and this sample protocol won't work for everyone. However, it will get you up and running until you can figure out your own groove. As I've mentioned, this book is about taking your health into your own hands; ultimately, it's up to you to decide what's most effective for you.

Wake up	Drink 12 ounces of water Exercise and/or meditate Take a cold shower or ice bath
Breakfast	Eat an anti-inflammatory breakfast
Mid-morning	Snack: anti-inflammatory smoothie
Lunch	Eat an anti-inflammatory lunch Walk for 10 minutes
Mid-afternoon (2–3 hours after lunch)	Snack: anti-inflammatory recipe from our cookbook
Dinner	Eat an anti-inflammatory dinner Walk for 10 minutes
Bedtime	No screens 1 hour before bed

LESS COMMON PROTOCOL

Infrared sauna	Two to four times a week 10–15 minute sessions, slowly up to 30–40 minutes
Alpha-Stim training	Daily
Hyperbaric oxygen therapy	Five days a week for 10–40 sessions total

FASTING WHILE ON THE INFLAMMATORY RESET

I typically suggest that people who are just beginning an anti-inflammatory diet start out by eating every two to three hours to help keep blood sugar levels stable. However, some people can comfortably fast right away and others cannot. In a nutshell, fasting should make you feel better, and you should be able to perform your usual daily activities easily and sleep well at night. If you can't, it's not for you.

THE BENEFITS OF FASTING WITH INFLAMMATION

If you can fast comfortably, doing so can increase your health dramatically. Research shows fasting can quickly and dramatically lower inflammation and improve your immune, gut, and brain health. In our clinics, we have many of our Hashimoto's and autoimmune patients undergo different types of fasts because we have found it is one of the surest ways to swiftly relieve their symptoms. These are some of the many benefits of fasting:

- Improved insulin sensitivity. Including periods of fasting in your daily routine has been shown to help cells become more insulin sensitive, which dampens the inflammation, metabolic imbalances, and brain degeneration caused by insulin resistance. One study found that restricting eating for a window of just eight hours each day significantly improved insulin resistance.

- Improved immune function. Intermittent fasting (for 12–18 hours each day) has been shown to improve immune function by reducing inflammation and minimizing the damage from inflammation. It also regulates immune function—great for autoimmune diseases—while regenerating immune cells and even lowering the risk of cancer.

- Improved brain function. Fasting and intermittent fasting reduces brain inflammation and supports brain repair. It also supports autophagy, or the removal of dead and dying cells in the brain, which will help your brain function more efficiently. Additionally, fasting boosts a brain chemical called brain-derived neurotrophic factor (BDNF), which protects your brain from neurodegenerative diseases such as Alzheimer's and Parkinson's.

- Improved cardiovascular function. Regular fasting can decrease "bad" cholesterol.

- Improved gut function. Fasting has been shown to lower inflammation in the gut and create a healthier composition of gut bacteria. And when you fast, the body switches from burning glucose for fuel to ketones that are stored in body fat. This is called **ketosis**, and it appears to reduce inflammation, support regeneration, and regulate metabolism.

WHEN YOU SHOULD NOT FAST

Fasting is not the quick route to better health. In our society, we are used to convenience and instant gratification, and people seek the same for their bodies, but that's not how fasting works.

While we have never had a patient feel worse from eating every two to three hours, we have had many patients feel much worse when fasting, especially coupled with any of the items listed here.

- Chronically low blood sugar
- Adrenal dysfunction
- Current or former brain injuries or other brain health challenges
- Diabetes medication
- Current or former eating disorders
- Pregnancy or trying to become pregnant

SMALL INTESTINAL BACTERIAL OVERGROWTH (SIBO)

When doing the Inflammatory Reset and changing diets, some people struggle with small intestinal bacterial overgrowth (SIBO) and must modify their 30-day reset to accommodate this gut dysfunction. As the name suggests, SIBO is a condition that arises from bacterial overgrowth in the small intestine. The small intestine does not typically harbor large populations of bacteria. However, in SIBO, bacteria migrate from the large intestine to the small intestine, where they ferment undigested food and produce gasses like hydrogen and methane. This can lead to digestive symptoms like bloating, gas, and abdominal pain, as well as health complaints like fatigue and joint pain.

Here are some symptoms of SIBO that may appear, particularly when you eat starches, some fruits or vegetables, or sugars:

- Abdominal bloating and distension
- Excessive gas (flatulence)
- Abdominal pain or discomfort, often in the lower abdomen
- Diarrhea or constipation (or alternating between the two)
- Fatigue and weakness
- Nausea or vomiting
- Weight loss (in some cases)
- Malnutrition or nutrient deficiencies
- Anemia (low red blood cell count)
- Joint pain or muscle pain
- Skin problems (such as acne or eczema)
- Headaches

THE INFLAMMATORY RESET

- Brain fog or difficulty concentrating
- Mood disorders (such as anxiety or depression)
- Food intolerances or sensitivities

Symptoms can vary in severity and may overlap with other gut disorders, so it's essential to take a SIBO test or experiment with your diet before coming to a definitive conclusion. If you feel bloated and gassy consistently, a good first step is seeing if you experience relief on a low-FODMAP diet, which reduces the carbohydrates and sugar alcohols that can cause bloating, pain, and more. If you ultimately have SIBO, you may have more success with the Inflammatory Reset by integrating the low-FODMAP guidelines.

Consult a health care provider for a breath test, the most well-regarded SIBO test, which tests for hydrogen and methane as byproducts of bacteria in the small intestine. While false negatives are common, a positive result means you have SIBO.

There are many ways to go about treating SIBO, but I recommend adopting a SIBO-specific Inflammatory Reset diet while taking antimicrobials for 30–60 days. The extended duration allows your body to adapt and change, and you can potentially feel the results.

RESETTING FOR 90 DAYS

You might be a little flabbergasted by the title of this section, as you're focused on the upcoming 30 days to reset your inflammation, but there are some incredible benefits in going for 90 days. In the first 30 days, when you cut out most foods and implement a variety of new exercises, your body is able to reduce your inflammation and perform better. But when you reach for two extra months, you allow your body to cement those habits and keep your inflammation down in the long term.

And in those two months, you can reintroduce foods—you know, the ones you can't live without—and see if they trigger your inflammation. The extra 60 days also allow you to integrate supplements, fasting, and even other exercises you were afraid to try (or eliminate those you don't want to do anymore!).

Finally, when you start the program, cutting things out of your diet might leave you feeling kind of crummy for seven to ten days. Some people find it's beneficial to go longer, ensuring they reach a place where they feel good with their dietary and exercise changes.

Whether you look at this as a time to tweak your inflammation plan or a continuation of the Inflammatory Reset, the added time is a second opportunity to take control of your inflammation and better mold the program to your life and liking.

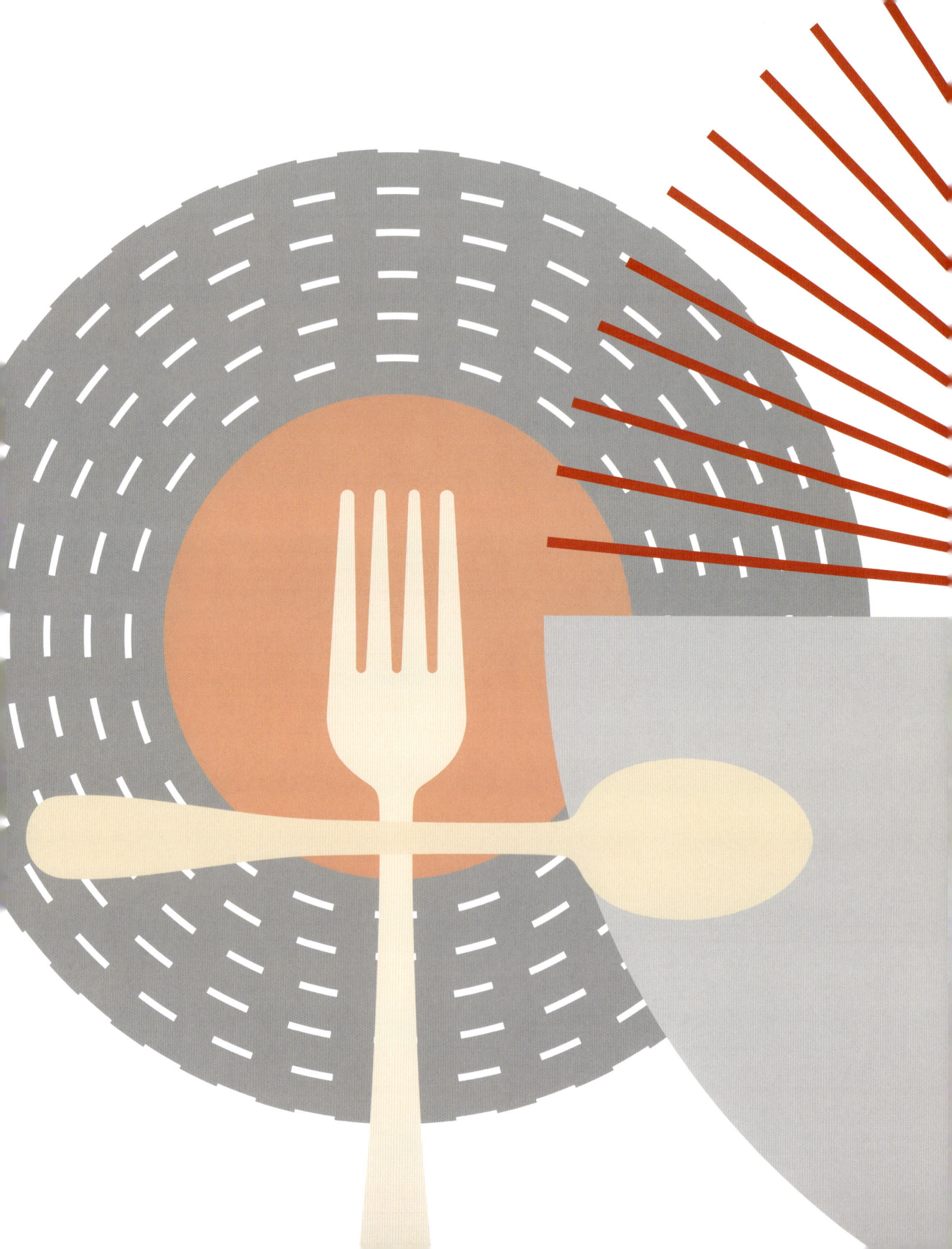

PART THREE

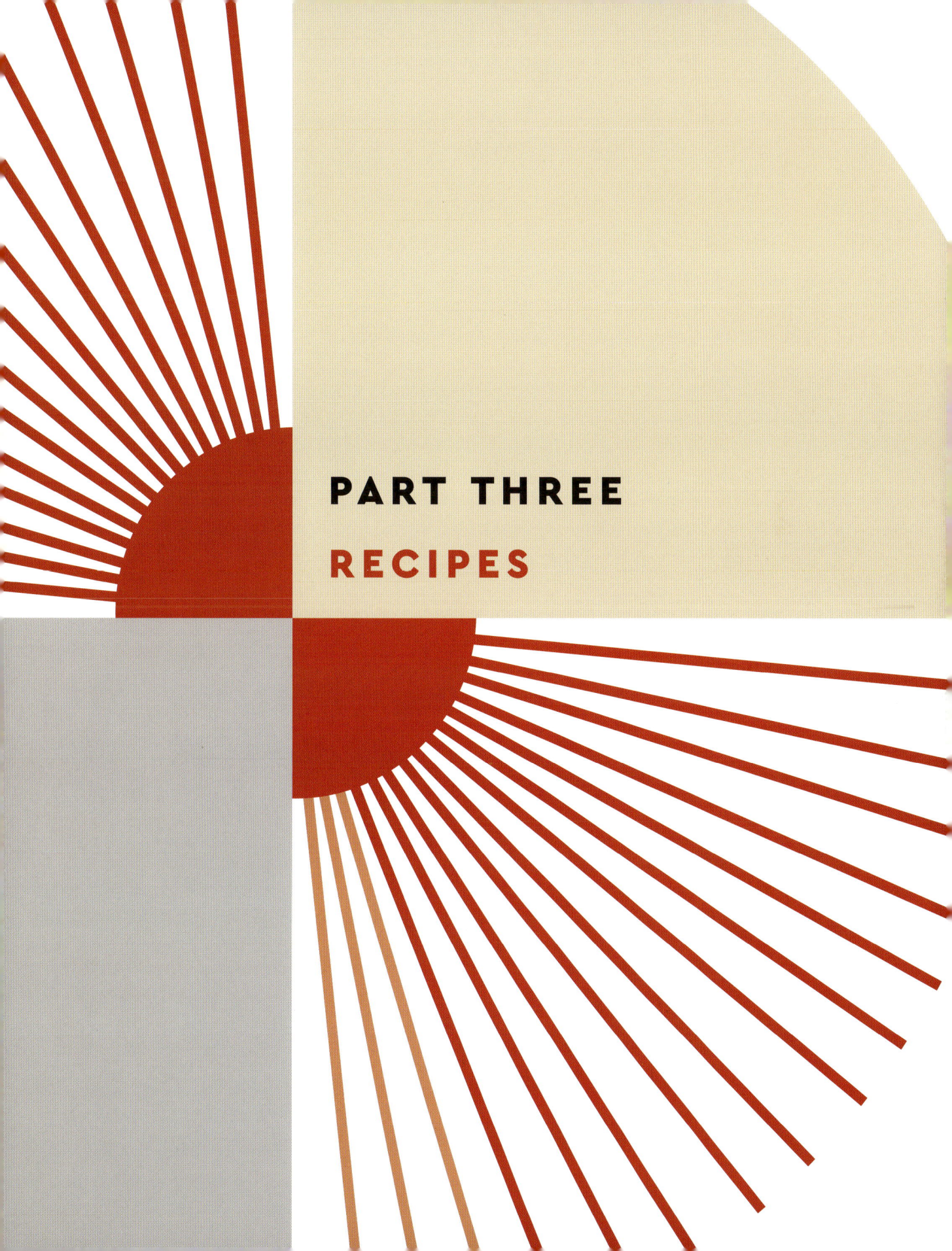

RECIPES

GETTING STARTED

A healthy diet is an essential part of the Inflammatory Reset, and in order to be successful, you need to commit to 30 days of eating anti-inflammatory foods and eliminating those that cause inflammation. This may seem restrictive, but you'll find that the recipes and kinds of foods you can make are a lot more appetizing than you might have anticipated.

These recipes are here to help you on your Inflammatory Reset journey, but you do not need to follow them exactly. Try experimenting with them! Add your own touches for your personal tastes. Ultimately, you want to feel comfortable in your kitchen cooking your own food.

You will notice that the Inflammatory Reset recipes exclude a lot of nightshades. Nightshades are a family of plants that include tomatoes, peppers, potatoes, eggplant, and some culinary spices, like paprika, black pepper, and cayenne pepper. The alkaloids in nightshades can trigger inflammation, so be sure to eliminate them if you know you are sensitive to them.

Another thing to consider is legumes. Although legumes are loaded with health benefits, some people are allergic to them or experience negative symptoms after consuming legumes. Some common kinds of legumes are peanuts and beans, including lentils, black beans, and garbanzo beans. If you have any negative symptoms after consuming legumes, discontinue eating them for the remainder of the Inflammatory Reset and retest them individually once you have completed the 30 days of elimination.

In addition to eating healthy foods, the Inflammatory Reset requires healthy eating habits. Like the exercises and activities in the protocol, eating is a behavior that you can adapt to make it healthier. Some basic guidelines:

1. Eat consistently and according to your appetite. Do not overeat—especially before bed—and don't let yourself go hungry.

2. Drink plenty of water. It's the building block of life, and therefore you need a lot. A good rule of thumb is to take your body weight, divide it in half, and

GETTING STARTED

drink that number of ounces. For example, someone who weighs 180 pounds needs to drink 90 ounces (about 3 quarts) of water.

3. Eat three meals a day, along with three small snacks at mid-morning, mid-afternoon, and before bedtime. This helps you feel sated and avoid overeating, along with balancing your blood sugar. During the 30 days of the Inflammatory Reset, your snacks will look a little different than usual. You can snack on any leftover approved meals or foods. You can also grab a handful of nuts with a small piece of fruit to keep it simple. Stick to the approved foods list and you can't go wrong; just be sure to include healthy fats and proteins to keep your blood sugar steady.

4. Make sure to eat vegetables and proteins for your three main meals. A balanced meal is everything, and you'll find many useful recipes in the following pages.

PRODUCTS TO MAKE YOUR RESET EASIER

Make this diet and any healthy diet a bit more doable by keeping a few products and snack foods on hand. Many of these items can be found at your local health food store or online at Thrive Market or Amazon. Remember to check that the ingredients in any prepackaged product are Inflammatory Reset friendly!

- Coconut wraps: add some nut butter or use as a sandwich wrap
- Collard green "wraps": use in place of any tortilla
- Seaweed wraps: add avocado and veggies for a quick snack
- Trail mix
- Cut-up vegetables in the refrigerator to grab as a snack
- Hummus or guacamole for a quick veggie dip
- Spiced nuts
- Apples or pears and nut butter
- Flax crackers
- Chickpea, black bean, or lentil pasta
- 100% buckwheat soba noodles

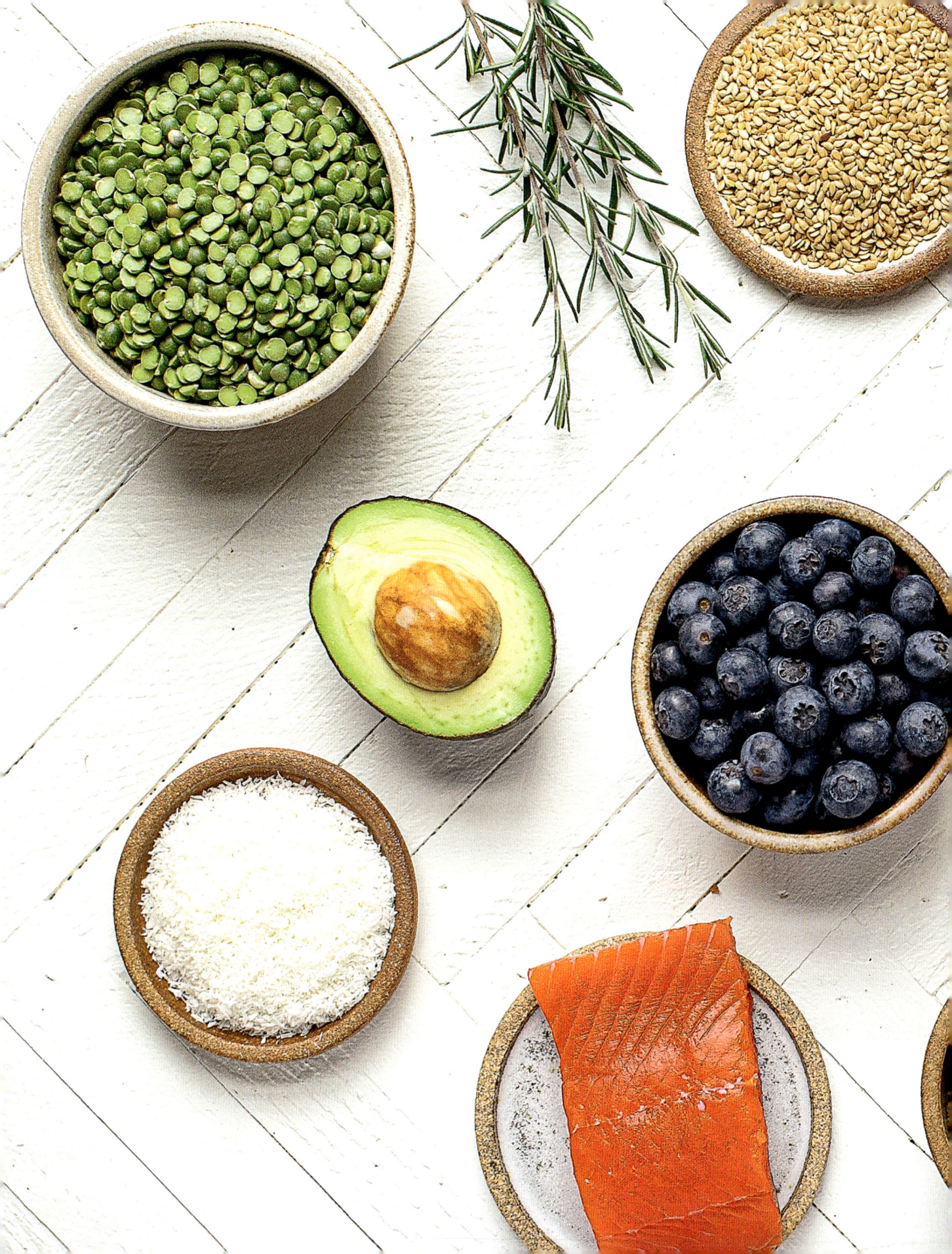

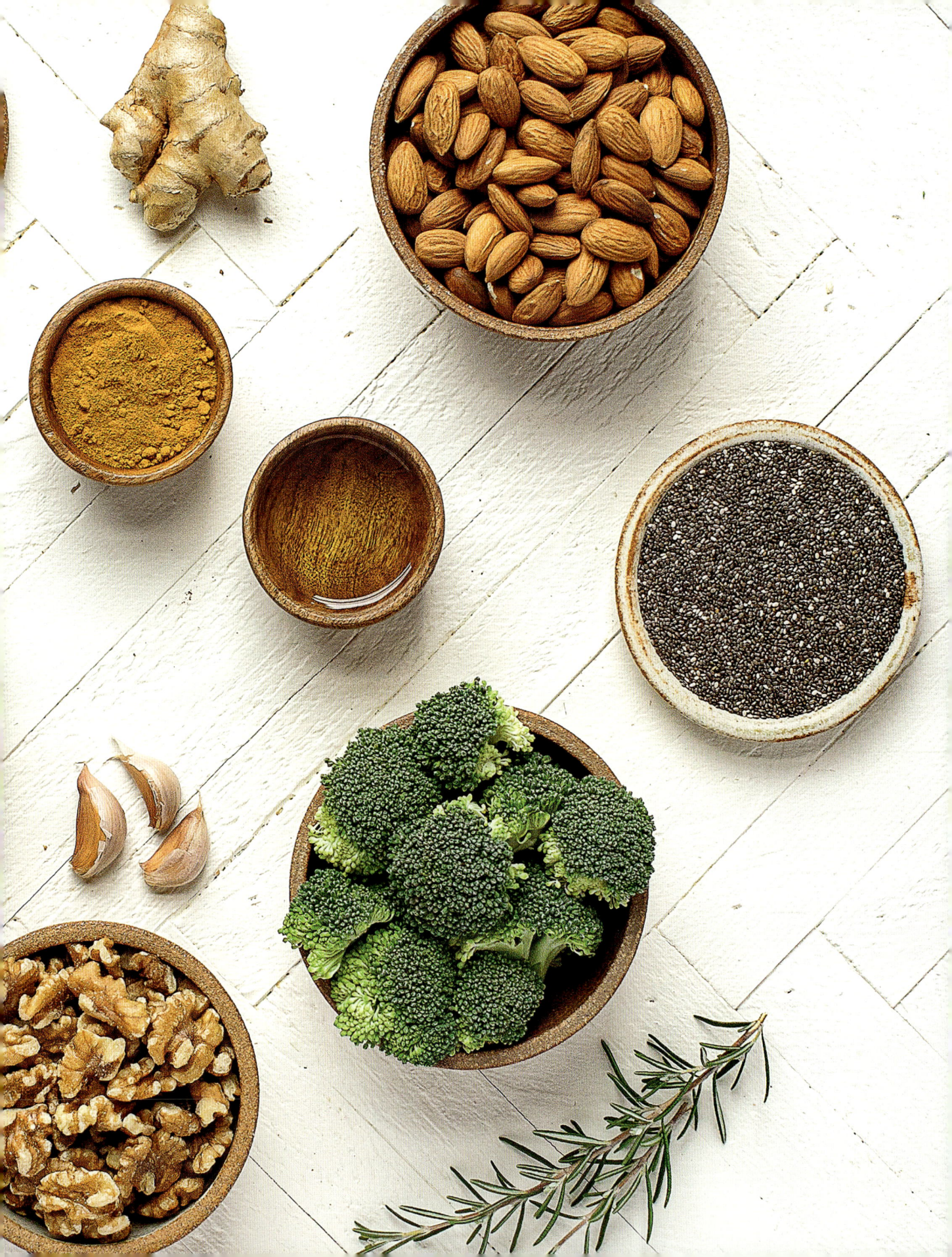

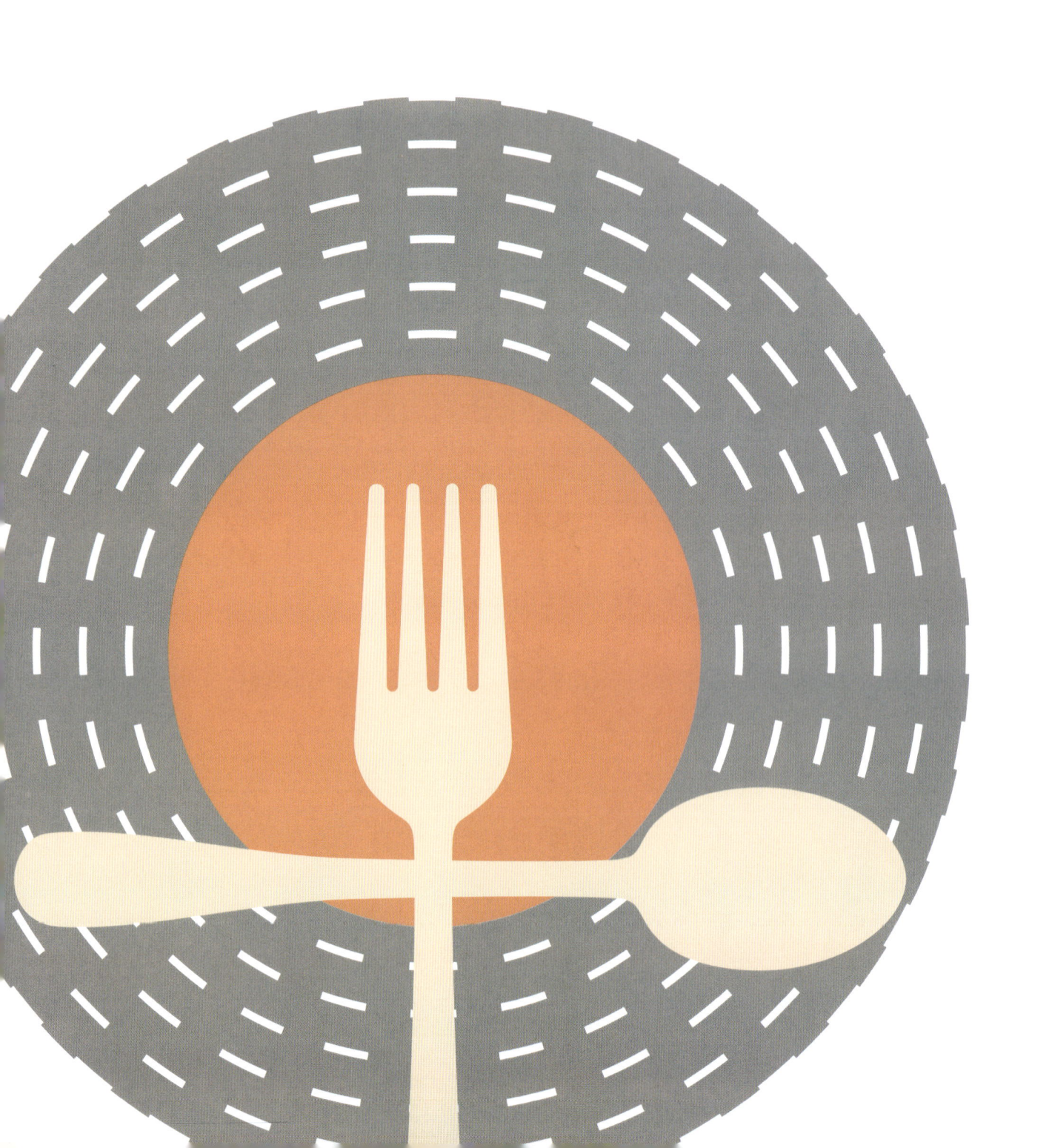

BREAKFAST

Starting the day with a healthy, antioxidant-rich, anti-inflammatory meal prepares each system in the body for a day of optimal functioning. We don't want to start the day with a blood sugar spike from eating foods high in sugar that trigger inflammation.

Every system of the body, from the immune system to the cardiovascular system to the gastrointestinal system, depends on the nutrients we choose to consume each day. Each recipe in the Inflammatory Reset offers a perfect balance of protein, fiber, and fat. There is something here for every day of the week, and you can enjoy expanding what breakfast looks like.

- Banana Buckwheat Pancakes
- Breakfast Turkey & Vegetable Hash
- Rosemary Root Vegetable & Kale Hash
- Morning Millet Cereal with Apple-Cinnamon Compote
- Apple-Cinnamon Breakfast Cobbler
- Cinnamon-Spiced Grain-Free Granola
- Berry Chia Pudding
- Golden Chai-Spiced Breakfast Porridge
- Homemade Turkey & Spinach Breakfast Sausage
- Golden Vanilla Chia Pudding

BANANA BUCKWHEAT PANCAKES

Great for a fun breakfast, these pancakes can be served with extra sliced bananas, shredded coconut, chopped nuts, or nut butter. Store leftover pancakes in the refrigerator for up to 4 days. Reheat in a toaster oven for a quick breakfast.

INGREDIENTS

1 cup buckwheat flour
1 tablespoon ground flaxseeds
1 teaspoon cinnamon
½ teaspoon baking soda
½ teaspoon sea salt
1 ripe banana
1 cup coconut or unsweetened almond milk
2 teaspoons apple cider vinegar
1 teaspoon vanilla extract
½ teaspoon lemon zest
1 tablespoon coconut oil

COOK TIME: 20 MINUTES
SERVES 6-8 PANCAKES

INSTRUCTIONS

1. In a large bowl, combine buckwheat flour, flaxseeds, cinnamon, baking soda, and salt.

2. In a separate bowl, mash banana. Add milk, apple cider vinegar, vanilla, and lemon zest and mix well.

3. Combine dry and wet ingredients together and mix well.

4. Allow batter to sit while you heat a medium-sized skillet on medium to medium-low heat.

5. Once skillet is hot, add coconut oil.

6. Drop pancake batter by the ¼ cup onto the hot skillet. Cook pancakes for 2–3 minutes or until they begin to bubble, then flip to other side for another 2–3 minutes.

7. Serve topped with creamy nut butter, sliced fruit, chopped nuts, or shredded coconut.

Buckwheat is a gluten-free seed grain—even though it has the word "wheat"—that is great for helping to keep blood glucose levels balanced, which is key in working to reduce inflammation. Most recipes made with buckwheat flour taste best when the buckwheat is freshly ground.

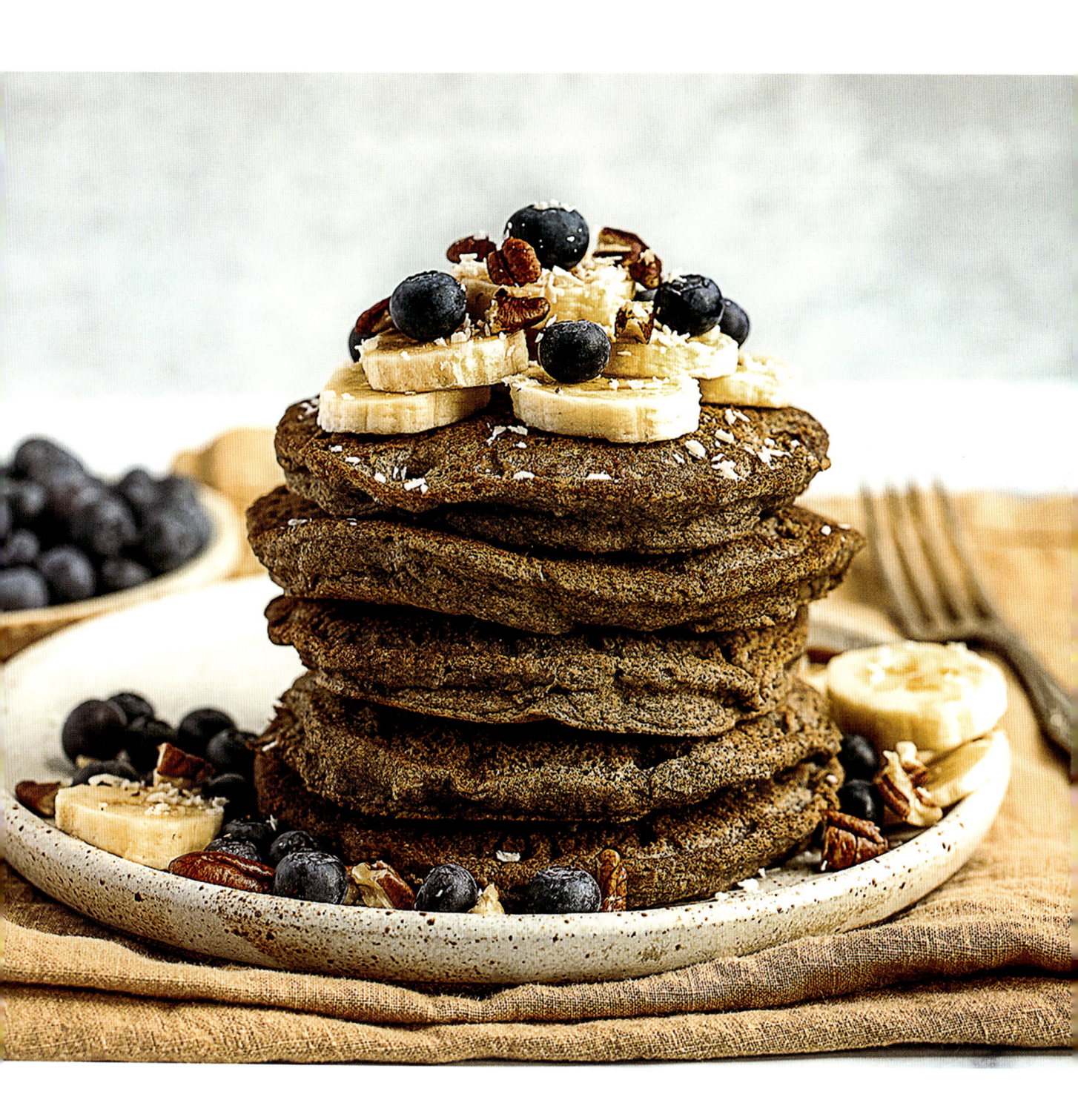

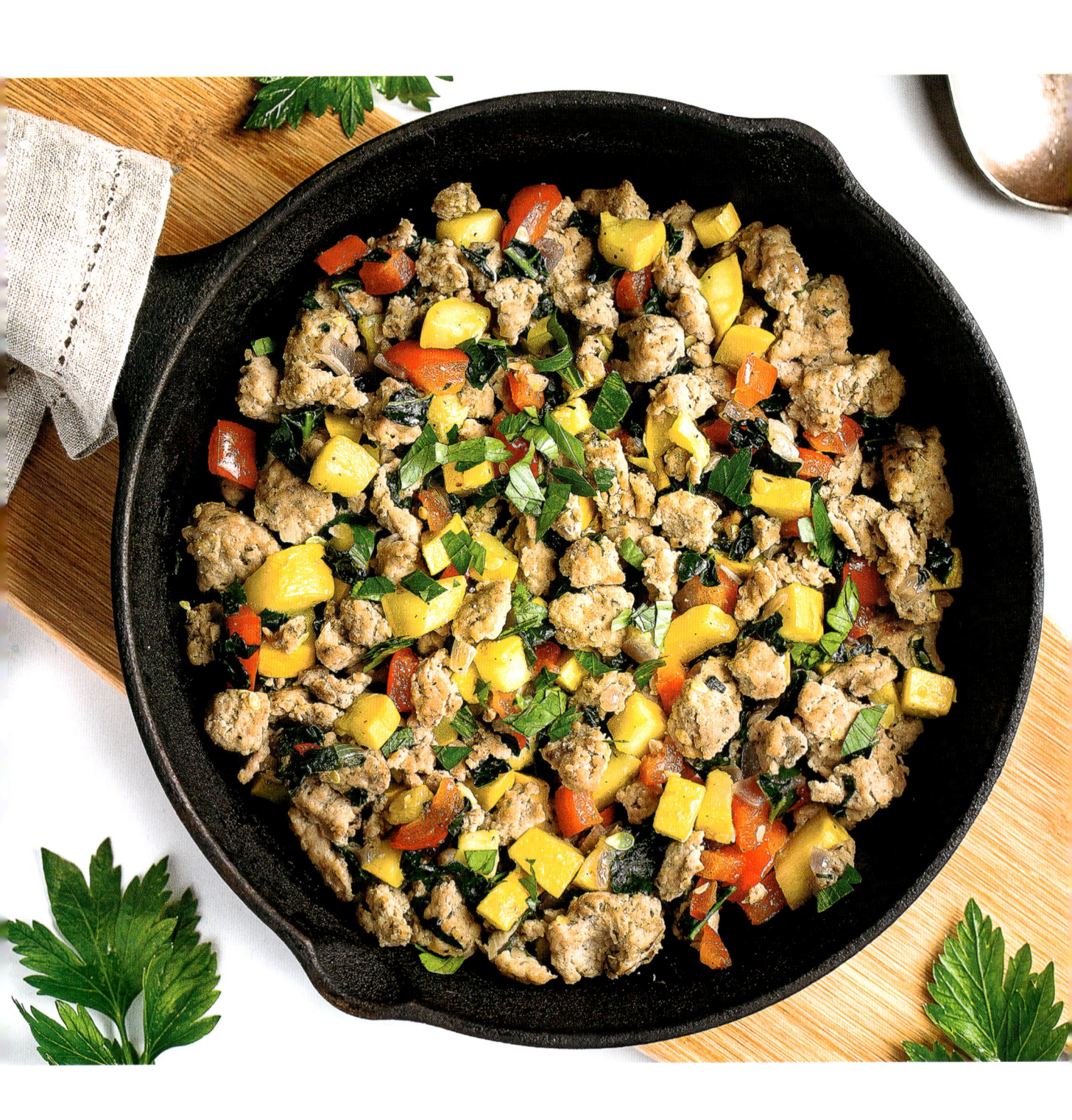

BREAKFAST TURKEY & VEGETABLE HASH

This breakfast hash can be made with ground turkey or ground chicken. Store it in the refrigerator in an airtight glass container for up to 4 days, and heat it up for a quick breakfast or snack. Use any combination of vegetables and herbs you prefer.

INGREDIENTS

- 1 pound ground turkey or chicken (preferably dark meat)
- 1 teaspoon sea salt
- 1 teaspoon dried thyme
- ½ teaspoon garlic powder
- ½ teaspoon sage powder
- Dash of pepper (optional; omit if nightshade-free)
- 3 tablespoons avocado or coconut oil, divided
- ½ red onion, chopped
- 1 zucchini or yellow summer squash, diced in ½-inch cubes
- ½ red bell pepper, diced (optional; omit if nightshade-free)
- 1–2 cups chopped greens (spinach, kale, chard)
- Additional salt and pepper to taste (omit pepper if nightshade-free)
- Fresh parsley for garnish (optional)

INSTRUCTIONS

1. Place ground turkey or chicken, salt, thyme, garlic powder, sage powder, and pepper in a large bowl. Combine the ingredients well and set aside.

2. Heat 2 tablespoons oil in a medium-sized cast-iron pan on medium heat. (Other pans work but not as well.)

3. Add red onion and a pinch of salt. Cook until soft and translucent.

4. Turn up heat to medium-high and add turkey. Stir frequently to break up meat until turkey is brown and cooked through, 5–7 minutes.

5. Push turkey mixture to the side of the pan and add the remaining 1 tablespoon oil, zucchini, red pepper, and a pinch of salt and pepper. Cook an additional 3–5 minutes until the zucchini is cooked through but not mushy. Add chopped greens and stir in until they turn bright green.

6. Combine turkey and vegetables. Cook an additional couple of minutes to combine flavors.

7. Adjust salt and pepper to taste and serve topped with chopped fresh parsley, if desired.

COOK TIME: 30 MINUTES
SERVES 4

ROSEMARY ROOT VEGETABLE & KALE HASH

This is a great alternative to a regular potato hash. Substitute any root vegetables or greens in place of the recipe ingredients. Substitute fresh or dried thyme for rosemary to your taste preference. You can also double this recipe and use the leftovers for a quick breakfast.

INGREDIENTS

- 1 medium turnip or celeriac root, peeled
- 1 carrot
- 1 parsnip, peeled
- 2 tablespoons avocado oil
- ½ red onion, chopped
- 2 garlic cloves, minced
- 1 tablespoon chopped fresh rosemary or 2 teaspoons dried
- ½ teaspoon sea salt
- Pinch of pepper (optional; omit if nightshade-free)
- ¼ cup water or broth
- 3 cups roughly chopped green kale
- Additional salt and pepper to taste (optional; omit pepper if nightshade-free)
- 2 tablespoons coconut aminos

INSTRUCTIONS

1. Dice the turnip or celeriac, carrot, and parsnip into ¼-inch pieces and set aside.

2. Heat a 12-inch pan or cast-iron skillet on medium heat and add oil.

3. Add red onion and a pinch of salt and cook until soft, 3–5 minutes.

4. Next, add garlic, diced turnips or celeriac, carrots, parsnips, rosemary, salt, and pepper. Cook for 3–5 minutes, stirring occasionally, until vegetables start to soften.

5. Add water or broth and reduce heat. Cover vegetables for 3–5 minutes or until soft and water has absorbed.

6. Remove the lid, add kale, and stir in. Raise heat to medium-high and cook an additional minute or so until kale wilts and all liquid is absorbed.

7. Turn off heat and season with salt, pepper, and coconut aminos to taste.

COOK TIME: 30 MINUTES
SERVES 4

> Whether you cook it fresh or dried, rosemary adds many medicinal benefits to your meals. Rosemary has a natural bitter taste that stimulates the gallbladder and liver to produce bile, a vital gastric secretion that breaks down the fats we eat.

MORNING MILLET CEREAL WITH APPLE-CINNAMON COMPOTE

This millet cereal is a great anti-inflammatory breakfast alternative to oatmeal. You can substitute berries, pears, or peaches for the apples and add a squeeze of lemon juice to brighten the flavor. Reduce the recipe by half for fewer people, or store leftovers in the refrigerator and reheat for a quick breakfast or snack.

INGREDIENTS

MILLET CEREAL
1½ cups millet
3 cups water
¼ teaspoon sea salt
Unsweetened coconut or almond milk

OPTIONAL
¼ teaspoon ground ginger
⅛ teaspoon ground nutmeg

OPTIONAL TOPPINGS
Hemp seeds
Chia seeds
Shredded coconut
Lemon juice

COMPOTE
1 tablespoon coconut oil
3 cups cored, peeled, and chopped apples
1 teaspoon ground cinnamon

INSTRUCTIONS

1. Heat a medium-sized pot on medium heat.

2. Add millet and stir for 3–5 minutes, or until it is toasty and golden brown.

3. Add water and salt. Bring to a boil, then lower heat to a simmer. Cover and cook for approximately 15 minutes. Turn off heat and allow millet to sit covered on the stove for 10 minutes.

4. While millet is cooking, add coconut oil to a small saucepan on medium heat. Add chopped apples, cinnamon, and optional spices and cook until apples are soft and fragrant.

5. When millet is done, remove the lid and fluff with a fork.

6. Scoop desired amount of millet into bowls, top with unsweetened coconut or almond milk, apple compote, and any optional toppings.

COOK TIME: 30 MINUTES
SERVES 4–6

> Millet, often thought of as a grain, is a seed that has a high fiber content and is very low on the glycemic index, which helps keep blood sugar in check. It is a good source of protein, antioxidants, zinc, iron, and calcium.

APPLE-CINNAMON BREAKFAST COBBLER

This apple cobbler is a wonderful fall or winter breakfast treat with no refined sugar, gluten, or grains. Feel free to use pears as a substitute and top it with unsweetened coconut yogurt if you'd like.

INGREDIENTS

FILLING

5–6 large Honeycrisp, Fuji, or any sweet red apple, peeled, sliced thin, cut into 1-inch pieces
Juice of ½ lemon
2–3 tablespoons melted coconut oil
1 teaspoon pumpkin pie spice
½ teaspoon sea salt

TOPPING

3 cups blanched almond flour
1 cup sliced almonds
¼ cup melted coconut oil
1 teaspoon cinnamon
1 teaspoon vanilla extract
½ teaspoon sea salt

INSTRUCTIONS

1. Preheat the oven to 350°F.

2. Add filling ingredients to a bowl and mix well. Transfer filling to a small casserole dish or square-shaped glass baking pan.

3. Mix all topping ingredients in a separate bowl and gently spread crumble on top of apples in an even layer.

4. Bake for 30–40 minutes until the top is a light golden brown and apples are soft.

5. Allow to cool for 15 minutes, then serve.

COOK TIME: 45–60 MINUTES

SERVES 4–6

> Cinnamon is one of the most health-promoting spices in our kitchen. Known for its antioxidant-rich polyphenols, cinnamon is great for reducing free radicals in the body. It is also considered one of the best foods for helping balance blood sugar levels in the body, making it a vital spice to bring into your Inflammatory Reset.

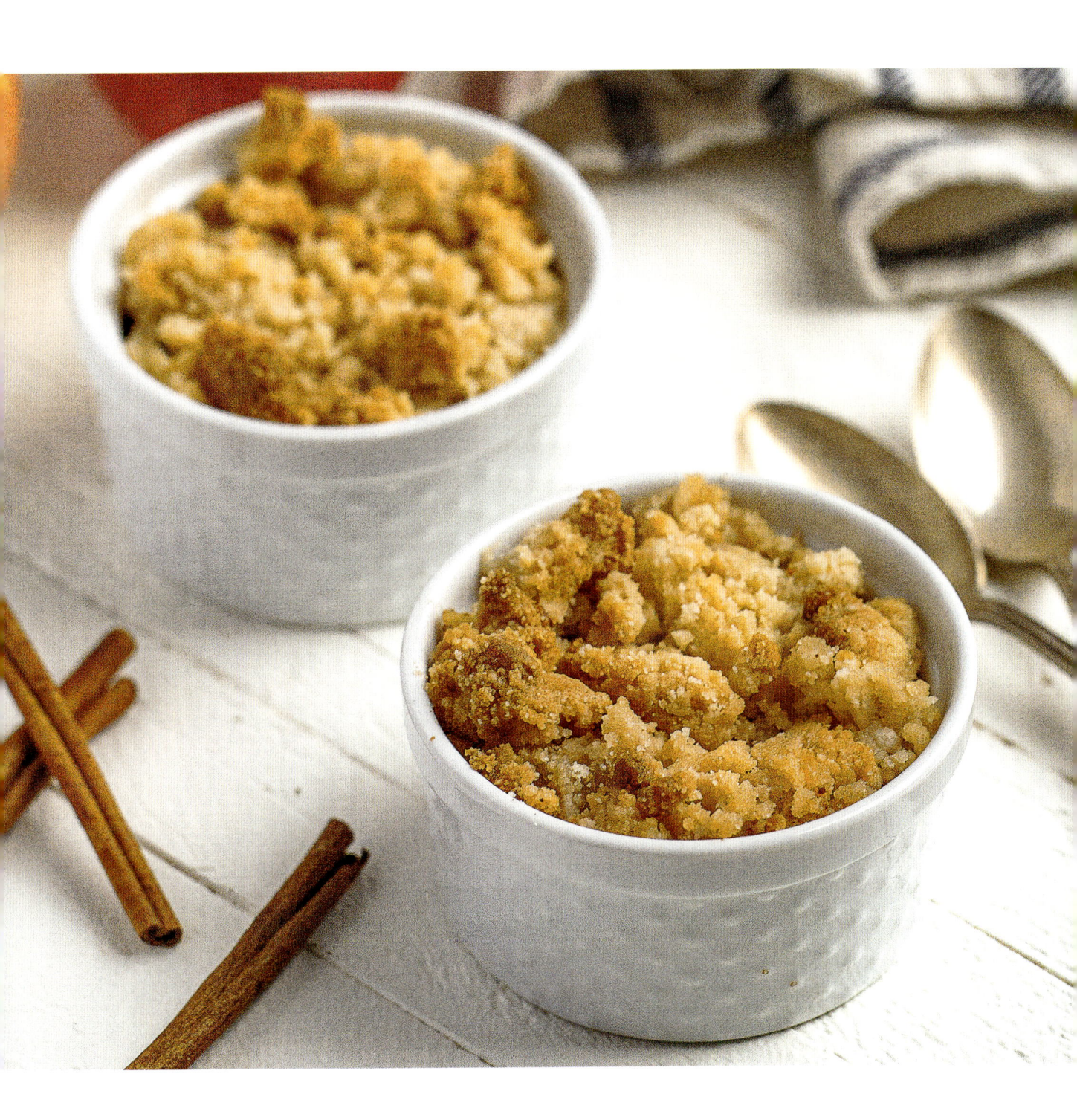

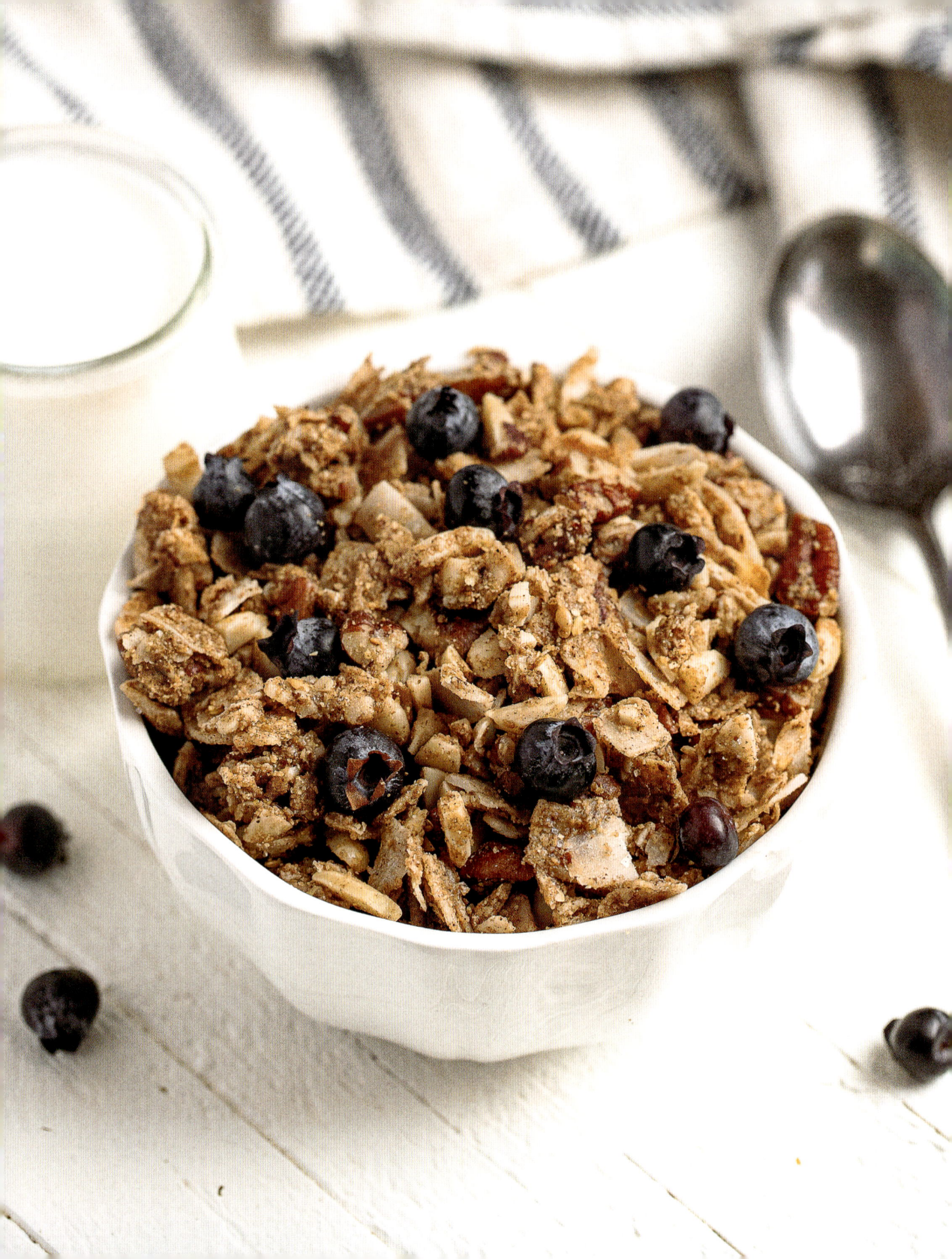

CINNAMON-SPICED GRAIN-FREE GRANOLA

This granola is great to have for a quick breakfast. Substitute any seeds for the nuts or ground chia seeds for flaxseeds. Store granola in an airtight glass container at room temperature for up to a week. Serve with your favorite nondairy milk and fresh blueberries, pears, apples, or strawberries.

INGREDIENTS

- 1 cup large coconut flakes
- ½ cup chopped pecans
- ½ cup chopped or slivered almonds
- ⅓ cup ground flaxseeds
- 1 teaspoon pumpkin pie spice or cinnamon
- ½ teaspoon sea salt
- 2 tablespoons melted coconut oil
- 1 tablespoon almond or cashew butter
- 1 teaspoon vanilla extract (optional)

INSTRUCTIONS

1. Preheat oven to 325°F.

2. Line an 8×8-inch pan with parchment paper.

3. Mix coconut flakes, pecans, almonds, ground flaxseeds, pumpkin pie spice or cinnamon, and sea salt together in a large bowl.

4. Mix oil, nut butter, and vanilla extract together in a separate bowl. Add this to the dry ingredients and mix until all ingredients are coated.

5. Press mixture flat in the lined pan.

6. Bake for 25–30 minutes or until golden brown.

7. Remove from oven and let cool in pan for an hour.

8. When cool, crumble granola completely into an airtight glass container for storage.

COOK TIME: 40 MINUTES
SERVES 6

BERRY CHIA PUDDING

This chia pudding can be made the night before and served as a breakfast or snack the next day. Use any kind of berry and, if full-fat coconut milk is unavailable, any unsweetened alternative milk.

INGREDIENTS

- 1 cup full-fat coconut milk (or any alternative milk)
- 1 cup fresh or defrosted frozen blueberries, strawberries, raspberries, or any combination
- ½ teaspoon lemon zest (optional)
- ¼ teaspoon vanilla extract
- Pinch of sea salt
- ⅓ cup chia seeds

OPTIONAL TOPPINGS
- Toasted coconut flakes
- Chopped nuts such as pecans, almonds, or cashews
- Berries

INSTRUCTIONS

1. Place coconut milk, berries, lemon zest, vanilla, and salt in a blender and blend until smooth.

2. Pour mixture in a medium-sized bowl and add chia seeds. Whisk until well combined.

3. Place chia pudding in an airtight glass container in the refrigerator for up to 3 hours or overnight.

4. Whisk or mix pudding before serving. Serve topped with chopped nuts, coconut flakes, and/or extra berries.

PREP TIME: 5 MINUTES
SET TIME: 3–4 HOURS
SERVES 2

> Chia seeds are an excellent source of alpha-linolenic acid (ALA), which is an omega-3 fatty acid. These omega-3s make chia an important addition to the Inflammatory Reset diet. Chia seeds have the potential to lower cholesterol levels, lower systemic inflammation, and help the body maintain balanced blood sugar levels.

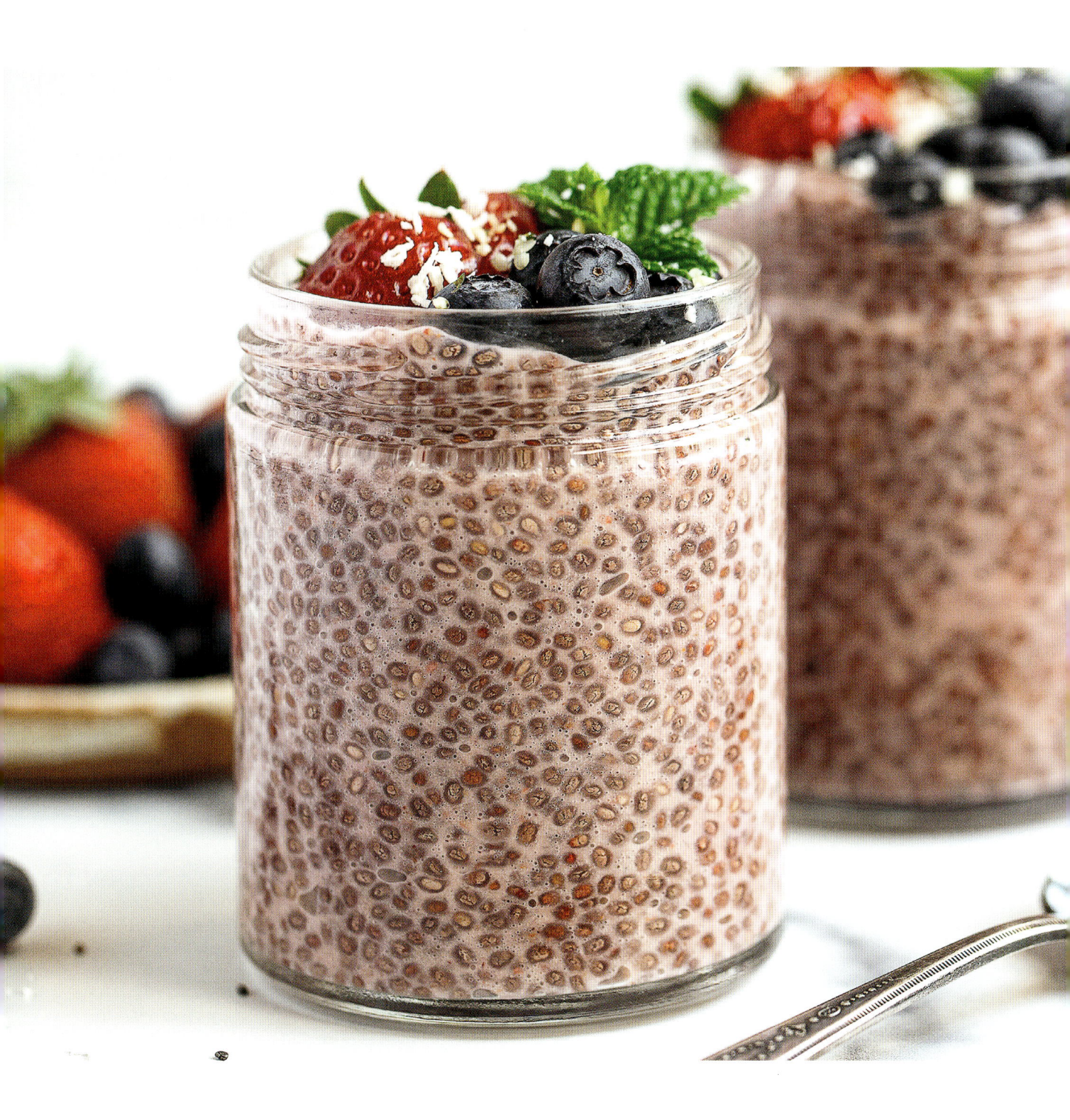

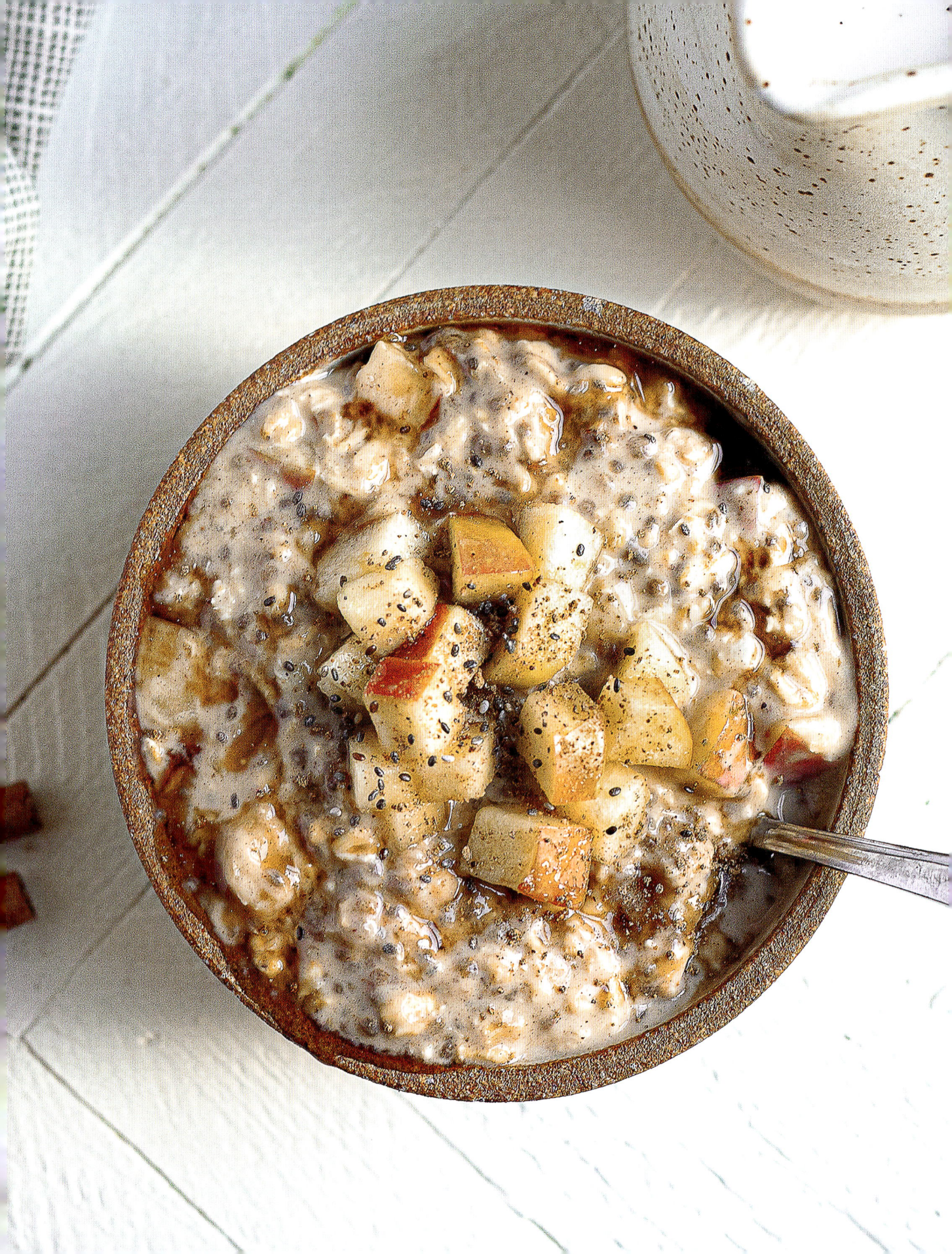

GOLDEN CHAI-SPICED BREAKFAST PORRIDGE

A great alternative to your traditional morning oatmeal, you can add any spices you like to this anti-inflammatory grain-free breakfast porridge and top it with freshly chopped apples, berries, or nuts. You can make a large batch of the dry ingredients (multiply by 4) and save it in your refrigerator. Just add warm almond or coconut milk for a quick morning breakfast.

INGREDIENTS

- ¼ cup finely shredded coconut
- 2 tablespoons almond flour
- 1 tablespoon ground flaxseeds
- 1 tablespoon chia seeds
- ¼ teaspoon cinnamon
- ⅛ teaspoon turmeric powder
- Pinch of cloves
- Pinch of black pepper (optional; omit if nightshade-free)
- 1 cup coconut or almond milk
- 1 teaspoon grated fresh ginger
- ¼ teaspoon vanilla extract
- ⅛ teaspoon sea salt

INSTRUCTIONS

1. Combine all dry ingredients except salt in a bowl.

2. Gently warm coconut or almond milk, ginger, vanilla, and salt in a small pot.

3. Add milk mixture to dry ingredients and stir well to combine.

4. Serve topped with fresh chopped berries, nuts, or apples, along with extra shredded coconut and a pinch of cinnamon if desired.

COOK TIME: 10 MINUTES
SERVES 1–2

HOMEMADE TURKEY & SPINACH BREAKFAST SAUSAGE

Serve these delicious breakfast sausages with a side salad and some steamed quinoa or millet. Store leftovers in the refrigerator for up to 4 days. Leftover sausages can be reheated and eaten any time of day. To reheat, simply cook on medium heat in a frying pan until hot.

INGREDIENTS

- 2 tablespoons avocado oil, divided
- 1 small yellow onion, chopped
- Pinch of sea salt
- 1 pound ground turkey or chicken (preferably dark meat)
- 2 cups chopped spinach
- 1 teaspoon sea salt
- 1 teaspoon dried thyme
- ½ teaspoon garlic powder
- ½ teaspoon sage powder

INSTRUCTIONS

1. Heat 1 tablespoon oil in a medium-sized pan or cast-iron skillet on medium heat. Add onions and a pinch of salt and cook until very soft, about 10 minutes. Set aside and let cool while preparing other ingredients.

2. Place ground turkey or chicken, spinach, salt, thyme, garlic powder, and sage powder in a large bowl along with cooked onions. Combine all ingredients well.

3. Heat the remaining tablespoon oil in a pan or cast-iron skillet on medium heat.

4. Form small-sized patties with sausage mixture and place in pan. Fry until golden brown, about 3–5 minutes. Flip and fry other side for another 2–3 minutes.

5. Feel free to serve sausages with a side of quinoa or millet and extra steamed greens or vegetables on the side. You can garnish with fresh parsley if you'd like.

COOK TIME: 30 MINUTES
SERVES 3–4

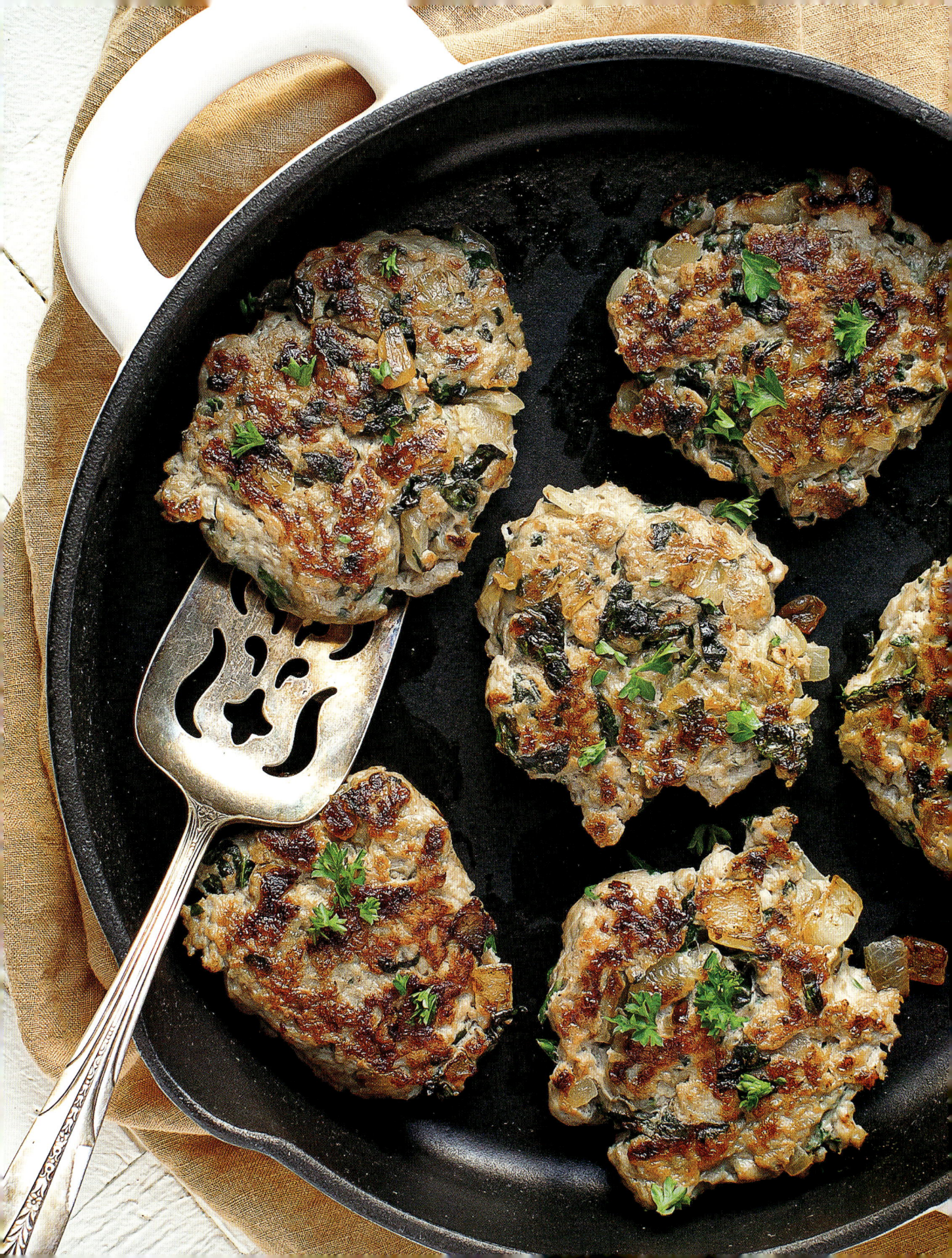

GOLDEN VANILLA CHIA PUDDING

Beyond breakfast, this chia pudding also makes a great dessert. You can top it with fresh berries, apples, pears, some cinnamon, or nutmeg. Store it in the refrigerator in an airtight glass container for up to 4 days.

INGREDIENTS

1 (13.5-ounce) can full-fat coconut milk

1 teaspoon vanilla extract

1 teaspoon lemon zest

½ teaspoon turmeric powder

Pinch of sea salt

¼ cup chia seeds

Chopped fresh fruit or berries (optional)

INSTRUCTIONS

1. Add coconut milk, vanilla, lemon zest, turmeric, and salt to a large bowl and whisk well.

2. Add chia seeds and whisk until well combined.

3. Pour the chia pudding into a jar or glass container and cover with a tight-fitting lid. Shake the jar, then refrigerate for 3 hours or overnight. Mix it once or twice while it is setting.

4. Feel free to top it with fresh seasonal fruit, shredded coconut, or spices of your choice.

PREP TIME: 5 MINUTES
SET TIME: 2 HOURS OR OVERNIGHT
SERVES 2

DRINKS & SMOOTHIES

A smoothie is one the best ways to consume a large amount of easy-to-digest vegetables. Think of it as a daily vehicle that ensures you get plenty of dark leafy greens, colorful nutrient-dense fruits, and fiber-rich vegetables into your diet. Use our smoothie recipes as a snack in between meals to keep your blood sugar regulated. Make one and store it in the refrigerator so that you can sip on it occasionally throughout the day.

- Strawberry-Banana, Chia & Almond Butter Smoothie
- Pineapple-Avocado Green Smoothie
- Creamy Coconut-Blueberry Smoothie
- Apple Pie Protein Smoothie
- Pumpkin Pie Protein Smoothie
- Cherry-Almond Smoothie
- Homemade Cashew Milk
- Apple, Ginger, & Cucumber Green Smoothie

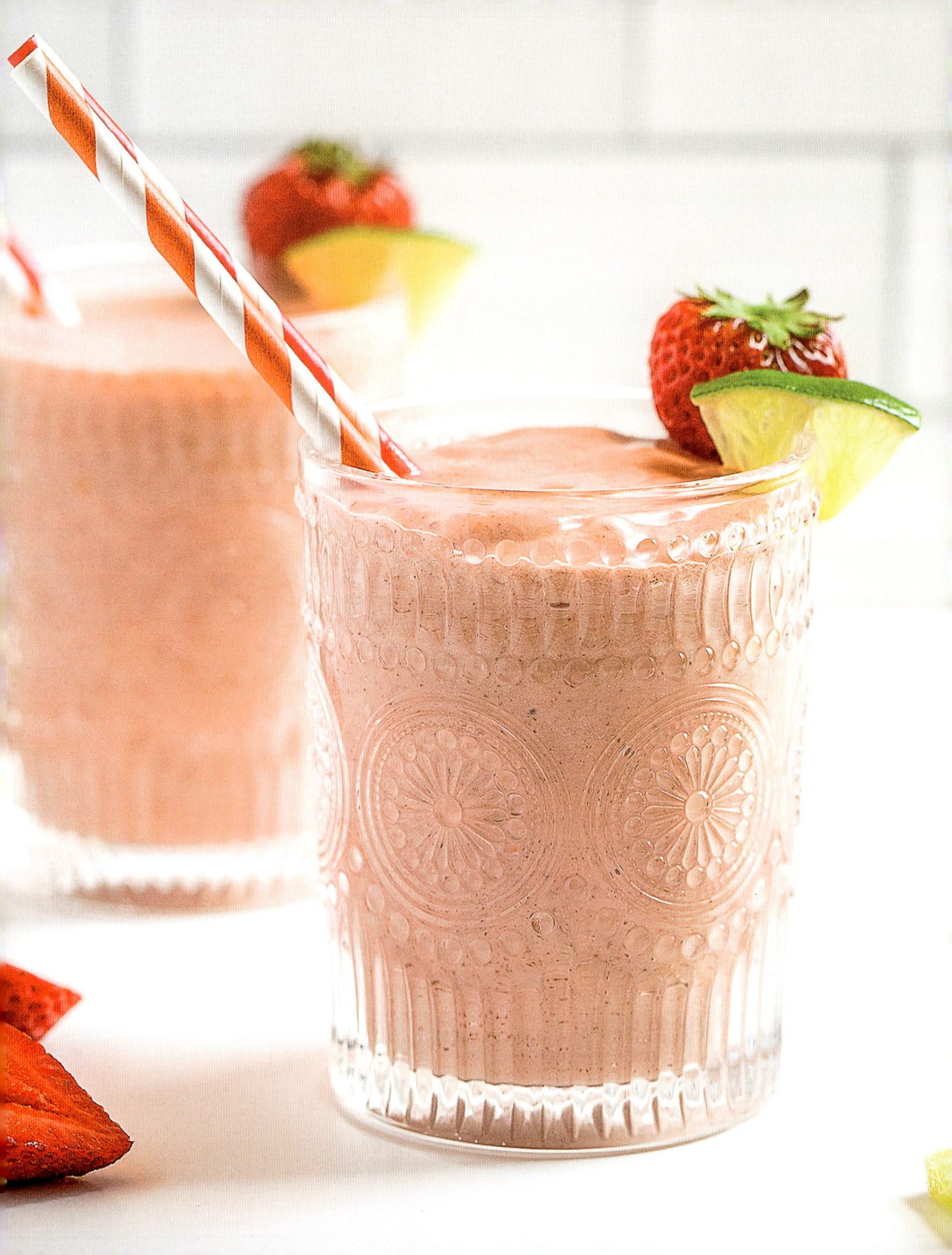

STRAWBERRY-BANANA, CHIA & ALMOND BUTTER SMOOTHIE

INGREDIENTS

2½ cups almond or coconut milk
2 cups frozen strawberries
1 frozen medium banana, sliced
2 tablespoons almond butter
1 tablespoon chia seeds
Pinch of sea salt
Squeeze of fresh lime or lemon (optional)

INSTRUCTIONS

1. Add all ingredients to a blender and blend until smooth.

PREP TIME: 5 MINUTES
SERVES 2-3

PINEAPPLE-AVOCADO GREEN SMOOTHIE

INGREDIENTS

2 cups coconut, almond, or alternative milk of choice
2 cups chopped kale leaves or packed baby spinach
2 cups frozen pineapple
1 medium frozen banana, sliced
½ medium fresh avocado, cut into pieces
¼ cup curly parsley leaves
2 tablespoons hemp seeds
Pinch of sea salt

INSTRUCTIONS

1. Add all ingredients to a blender and blend until smooth.

PREP TIME: 10 MINUTES
SERVES 2

Avocados are considered one of the world's healthiest foods for a reason. For starters, they are a simple, delicious fat that is easy to digest, and they are very high in fiber, making them a superfood for the digestive system. Avocados are also high in monounsaturated fats, which make them highly beneficial to your heart and brain health. They also have the potential to improve fasting insulin levels, which helps protect the body from insulin resistance and diabetes. Add to the mix of health benefits all the potassium, vitamin K, folate, and vitamin C that avocados are chock-full of, and you get a clear picture as to why avocados are a great addition to smoothies like these!

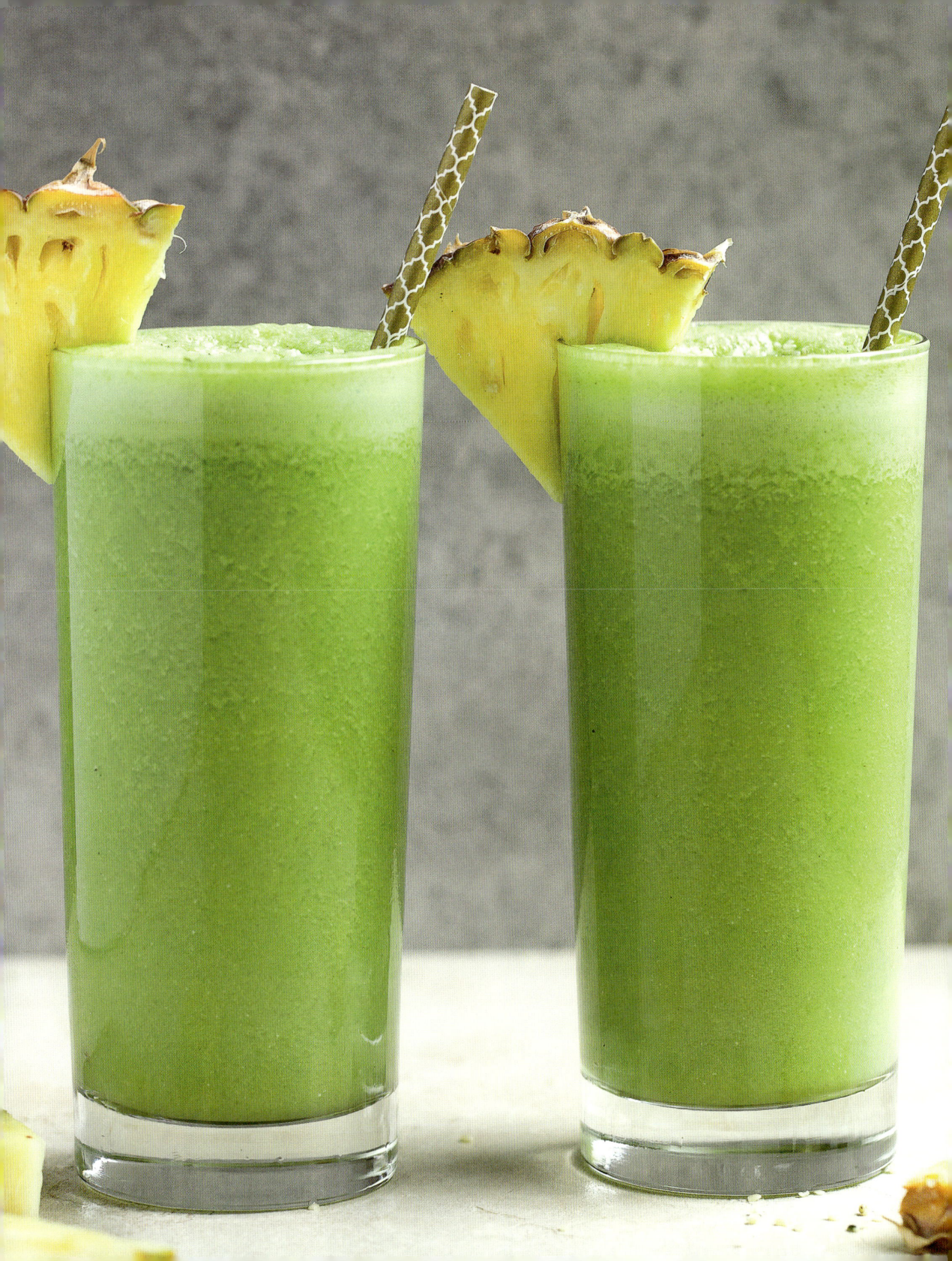

CREAMY COCONUT-BLUEBERRY SMOOTHIE

INGREDIENTS

3 cups coconut milk
2 cups frozen blueberries
½ fresh or frozen banana, sliced
1 tablespoon chia seeds
1 teaspoon lemon zest
½ teaspoon vanilla extract
Pinch of sea salt
1 scoop anti-inflammatory protein powder (optional)

INSTRUCTIONS

1. Add all ingredients to a blender and blend until smooth.

PREP TIME: 5 MINUTES
SERVES 2

> Blueberries are one of the most antioxidant-rich and nutrient-dense fruits we can eat. They are known to have significant anti-inflammatory effects on the body, are high in fiber, and promote regularity and the health of the digestive tract.

APPLE PIE PROTEIN SMOOTHIE

This apple pie smoothie is a delicious fall breakfast or snack. You can throw in a handful of greens, your favorite Inflammatory Reset–friendly protein powder, or a scoop of hemp seeds. If you like the flavor of ginger, you can add more for a spicier smoothie.

INGREDIENTS

2 cups unsweetened coconut or almond milk
1 medium apple, loosely chopped
1 large frozen banana, sliced
1 tablespoon almond butter
1 tablespoon chia seeds
1 teaspoon cinnamon
1 teaspoon grated fresh ginger or a pinch of ginger powder
½ teaspoon vanilla extract
Pinch of sea salt

INSTRUCTIONS

1. Add all ingredients to a blender and blend until smooth.

PREP TIME: 5 MINUTES
SERVES 2

> Apples have a soluble fiber in them called pectin, which binds to toxins and excess cholesterol in the gastrointestinal tract, promoting both detoxification and elimination. Apples are also high in antioxidants, making them a superfood for the Inflammatory Reset diet.

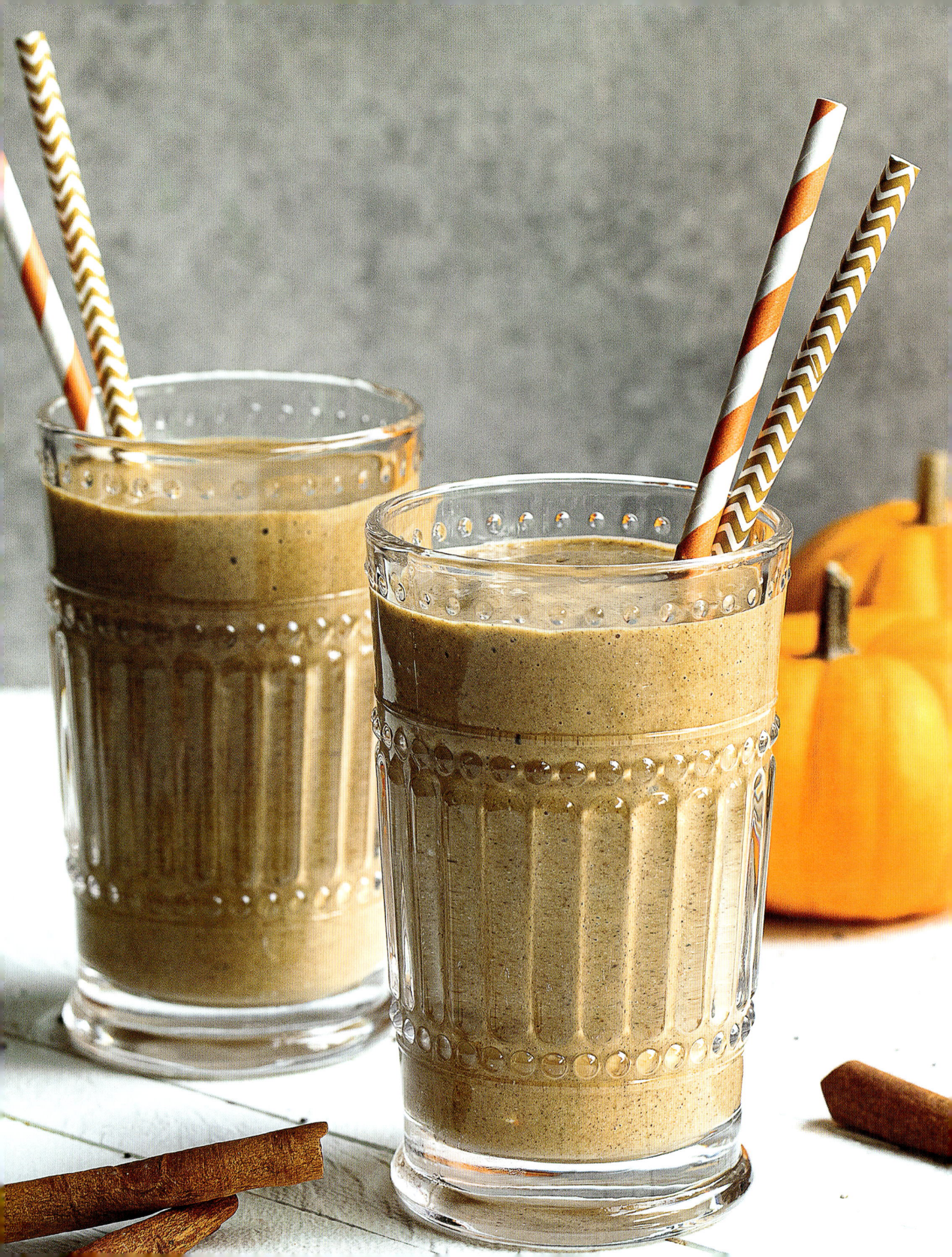

PUMPKIN PIE PROTEIN SMOOTHIE

This smoothie is a delicious protein-packed treat. You can add more ginger or cinnamon if you like more spice. You can also substitute pumpkin pie spice for the cinnamon. Add extra almond butter or chia seeds for more protein.

INGREDIENTS

1½ cups almond or coconut milk
1½ frozen bananas, sliced
1 cup ice
½ cup organic pumpkin puree
2 tablespoons almond butter
1–2 teaspoons grated fresh ginger or a pinch of ginger powder
1 tablespoon chia seeds
1 teaspoon cinnamon
1 teaspoon lemon zest
½ teaspoon vanilla extract
Pinch of sea salt

INSTRUCTIONS

1. Add all ingredients to a blender and blend until smooth.

PREP TIME: 5 MINUTES
SERVES 2

CHERRY-ALMOND SMOOTHIE

This tart smoothie makes a great breakfast or post-workout snack. You can use any nut butter you like; try cashew butter or pecan butter for a sweeter smoothie.

INGREDIENTS

2 cups almond or coconut milk
1½ cups frozen cherries
½–1 frozen banana
2 tablespoons almond butter
2 tablespoons chia seeds
½ teaspoon almond or vanilla extract (optional)
Pinch of sea salt

INSTRUCTIONS

1. Add all ingredients to a blender and blend until smooth.

PREP TIME: 5 MINUTES
SERVES 2

> Cherries are a potent source of anthocyanins, which are what give cherries their deep red color. These antioxidant-rich, cancer-fighting polyphenols help the body ward off oxidative stress while at the same time increasing the amount of vitamin C you consume.

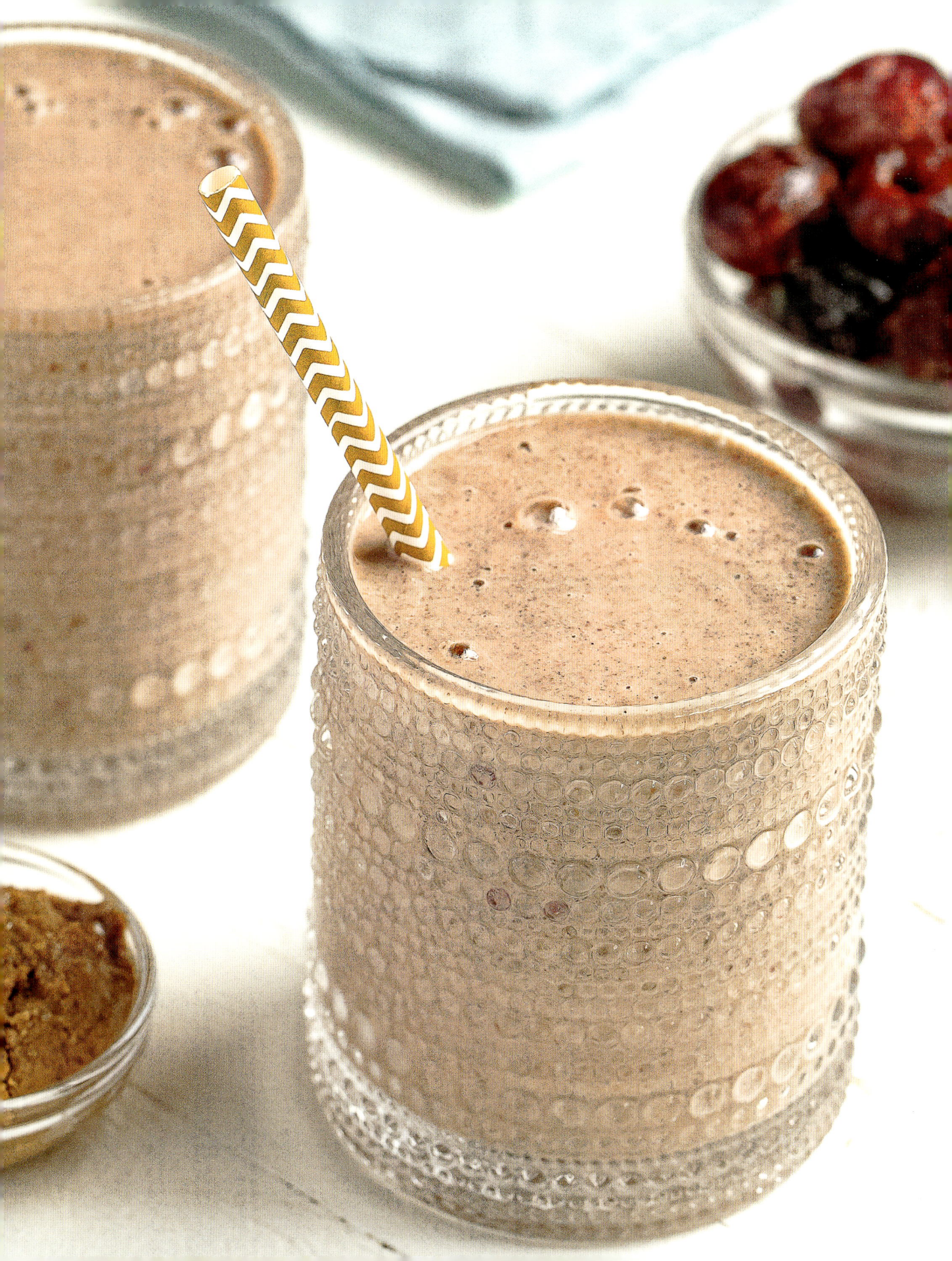

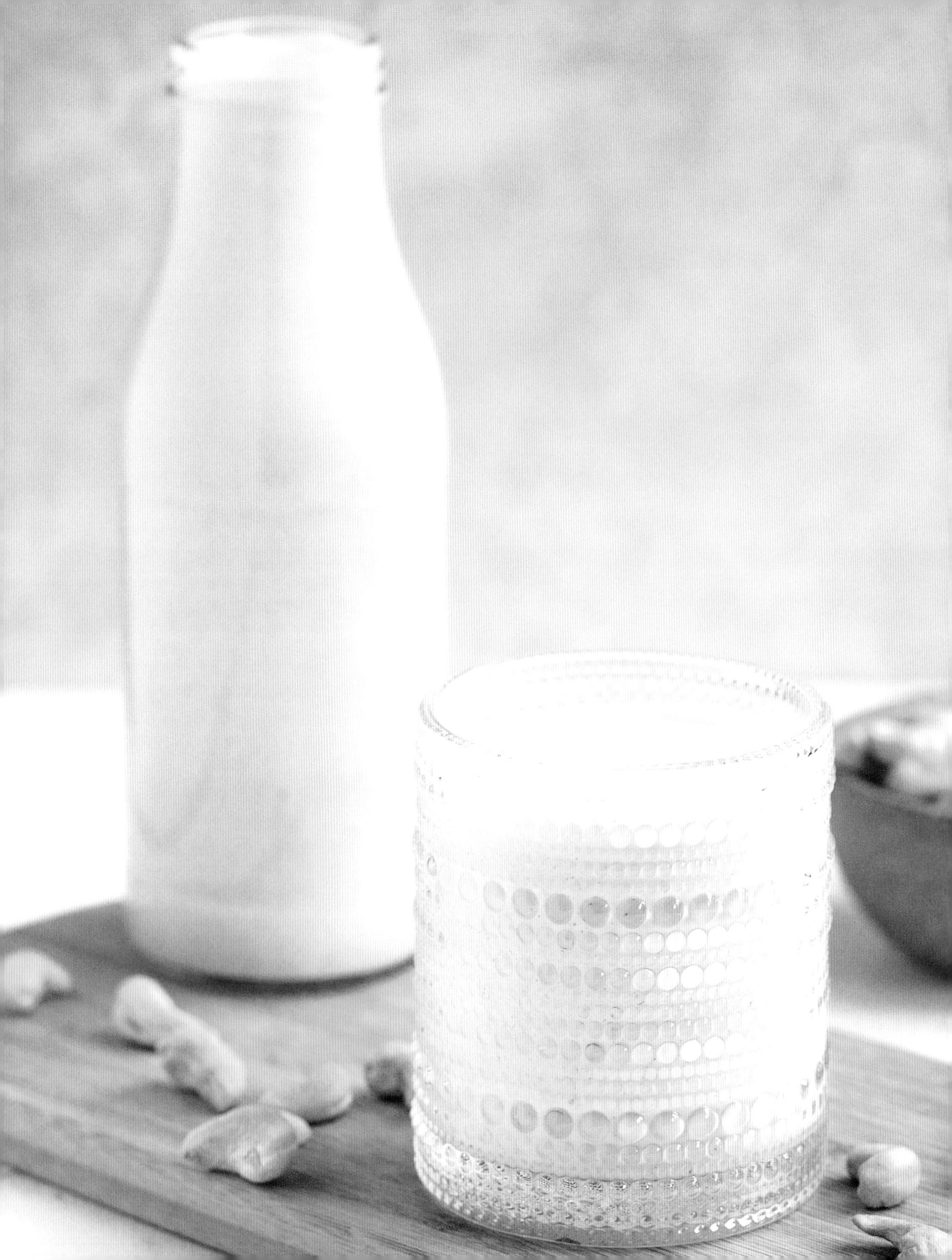

HOMEMADE CASHEW MILK

Of all of the nut milks, cashew milk is the easiest to make. If you soak cashews before blending them in a high-speed blender, such as a Vitamix or Blendtec, there is no need to strain the mixture; it simply blends right in. Add extra cinnamon or other herbs such as cardamom or ginger if you'd like more spice. Store in an airtight glass container in the refrigerator for up to a week.

INGREDIENTS

1 cup raw cashews
4 cups water
1 teaspoon vanilla extract
¼ teaspoon cinnamon (optional)
Pinch of sea salt

INSTRUCTIONS

1. Soak cashews in cold water for 4–8 hours or overnight. Alternatively, if you are short on time you can soak them in hot water for 30 minutes then strain and rinse cashews well.

2. Add them with all other ingredients to a high-speed blender and blend until smooth.

SOAK TIME: 30 MINUTES TO OVERNIGHT
PREP TIME: 5 MINUTES
SERVES 4

APPLE-GINGER-CUCUMBER GREEN SMOOTHIE

INGREDIENTS

2 cups coconut or almond milk
2 cups baby spinach leaves or other chopped greens
1 apple, loosely chopped
½ frozen banana, sliced
½ medium cucumber, sliced
2 tablespoons hemp or chia seeds
1 teaspoon grated fresh ginger
1 teaspoon lemon zest (optional)
Pinch of sea salt

INSTRUCTIONS

1. Add all ingredients to a blender and blend until smooth.

PREP TIME: 5 MINUTES
SERVES 2

Ginger is an antioxidant-rich culinary spice that helps fight inflammation in the gastrointestinal tract. Reducing inflammation in the gut is a key first step in healing inflammation in the body. Ginger can be added to smoothies, juices, soups, curries, and stir-fries, which makes it easy to get a daily dose of this anti-inflammatory spice in your food.

SIDES, SNACKS & SALADS

Remember that snacks for these 30 days will look a little different, so be sure to use any of these sides, snacks, and salads as a "snack" to balance your blood sugar during your Inflammatory Reset. The recipes are void of all processed foods and will not only help to maintain your blood sugar levels and keep you satiated, but also keep your taste buds happy.

- Asian Chicken Salad with Fresh Herbs
- Chicken Caesar Salad
- Crunchy Mediterranean Salmon Salad
- Roasted Sweet Potato, Quinoa & Kale Salad
- Roasted Vegetable & Kale Salad with Apple Cider Vinaigrette
- Snap Pea, Radish & Mint Salad
- Rainbow-Cabbage Fennel Slaw
- Wild Salmon Salad
- Apple & Nut Butter Chia Boats
- Everything Almond Crackers
- Curry Spiced Nuts
- Easy Oven-Baked Kale Chips
- Creamy Dairy-Free Spinach-Artichoke Dip
- Easy Chickpea Socca

ASIAN CHICKEN SALAD WITH FRESH HERBS

This chicken salad is a delicious light meal that's simple to make. You can bake the chicken breasts ahead of time and store them in the refrigerator so it's easy to throw the salad together for a quick lunch or snack. Add extra herbs, lime, and salt and pepper to taste.

INGREDIENTS

- 1 medium boneless, skinless chicken breast
- Sea salt and pepper (omit pepper if nightshade-free)
- ¼ cup lime juice
- ¼ cup avocado oil
- 4 teaspoons coconut aminos
- 1 teaspoon lime zest
- 1 medium napa cabbage sliced very thin, about 7 cups
- 1 red pepper, cut into matchsticks (optional; omit if nightshade-free)
- ½ cup chopped fresh basil
- ½ cup chopped fresh cilantro
- 2 green onions, sliced thin

INSTRUCTIONS

BAKED CHICKEN INSTRUCTIONS

1. Preheat oven to 350°F.

2. Place chicken breast in a glass baking dish and sprinkle generously with sea salt and pepper.

3. Bake for 1 hour.

4. Remove and let cool.

5. Cut into bite-sized cubes or pieces and set aside.

SALAD INSTRUCTIONS

1. Whisk lime juice, oil, coconut aminos, and lime zest together in a large bowl.

2. Add cabbage, bell pepper, basil, cilantro, and green onions. Toss to combine.

3. Fold in chicken, sprinkle with an extra ¼–½ teaspoon sea salt and pepper to taste.

> Cilantro is an antioxidant-rich herb that has many medicinal properties as well. It plays into your Inflammatory Reset with its ability to help rid the body of heavy metals by binding to them in the tissue, which allows the body to excrete them via the stool.

COOK TIME: 1 HOUR FOR CHICKEN
PREP TIME: 10 MINUTES
SERVES 4

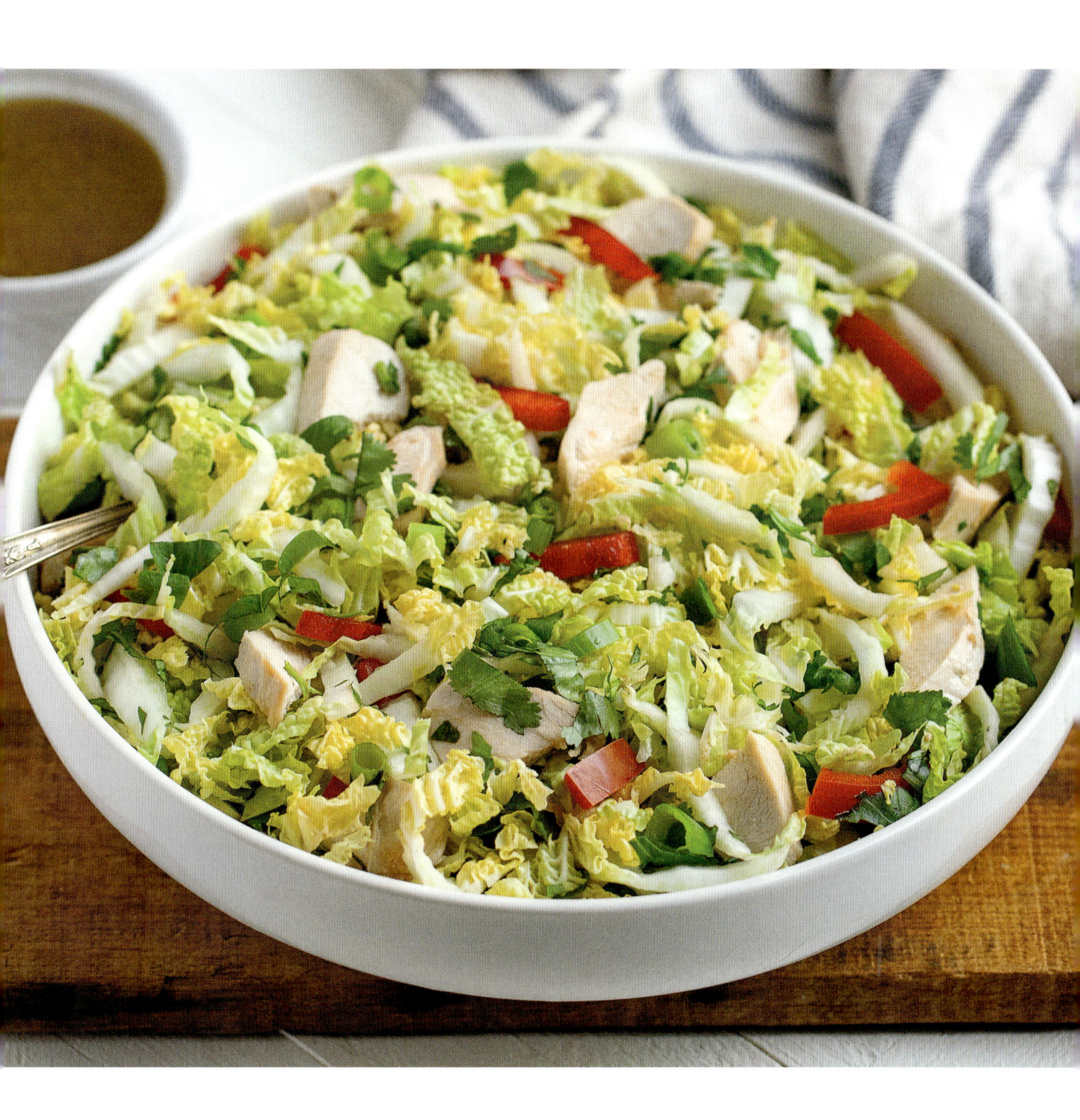

CHICKEN CAESAR SALAD

This great dairy-free Caesar salad has a dressing that is loaded with healthy ingredients. For a different protein, try grilled grass-fed lamb, albacore tuna, or salmon. Store any leftover dressing in the refrigerator for up to a week.

INGREDIENTS

SALAD

1 large head of romaine lettuce, chopped

2 cups cubed cooked chicken breast (or other protein)

DRESSING

½ cup water

½ cup olive oil

2 ribs celery, chopped

Juice of ½ lemon

3–4 tablespoons coconut aminos

1 tablespoon dulse flakes

1 garlic clove, minced

INSTRUCTIONS

1. Add all salad dressing ingredients to a blender and blend until smooth and creamy.

2. Toss desired amount of dressing with chopped romaine. You can add extra dressing to individual bowls.

3. Serve topped with cubed chicken and an extra squeeze of lemon if desired.

PREP TIME: 15 MINUTES
SERVES 3–4

CRUNCHY MEDITERRANEAN SALMON SALAD

Loaded with prebiotics and healthy fats, this delicious salad can be enjoyed as a quick snack or wrapped in lettuce leaves with avocado and sliced green onions for an easy lunch. Store in the refrigerator for up to 3 days.

INGREDIENTS

- 2 (6-ounce) cans wild-caught salmon, drained
- 3 celery sticks chopped
- ½ large cucumber, seeded and chopped
- ½ cup kalamata olives
- ½ cup chopped artichoke hearts
- ½ cup chopped fresh cilantro or parsley
- 2 tablespoons olive oil
- 2 tablespoons lemon juice
- ¼–½ teaspoon sea salt
- Fresh romaine lettuce leaves, chopped into bite-size pieces
- Chopped avocado (optional)
- Sliced green onions (optional)

INSTRUCTIONS

1. Add all ingredients to a large bowl and mix well until combined.

2. Add extra salt, lemon juice, or fresh herbs to taste.

PREP TIME: 15 MINUTES
SERVES 4–6

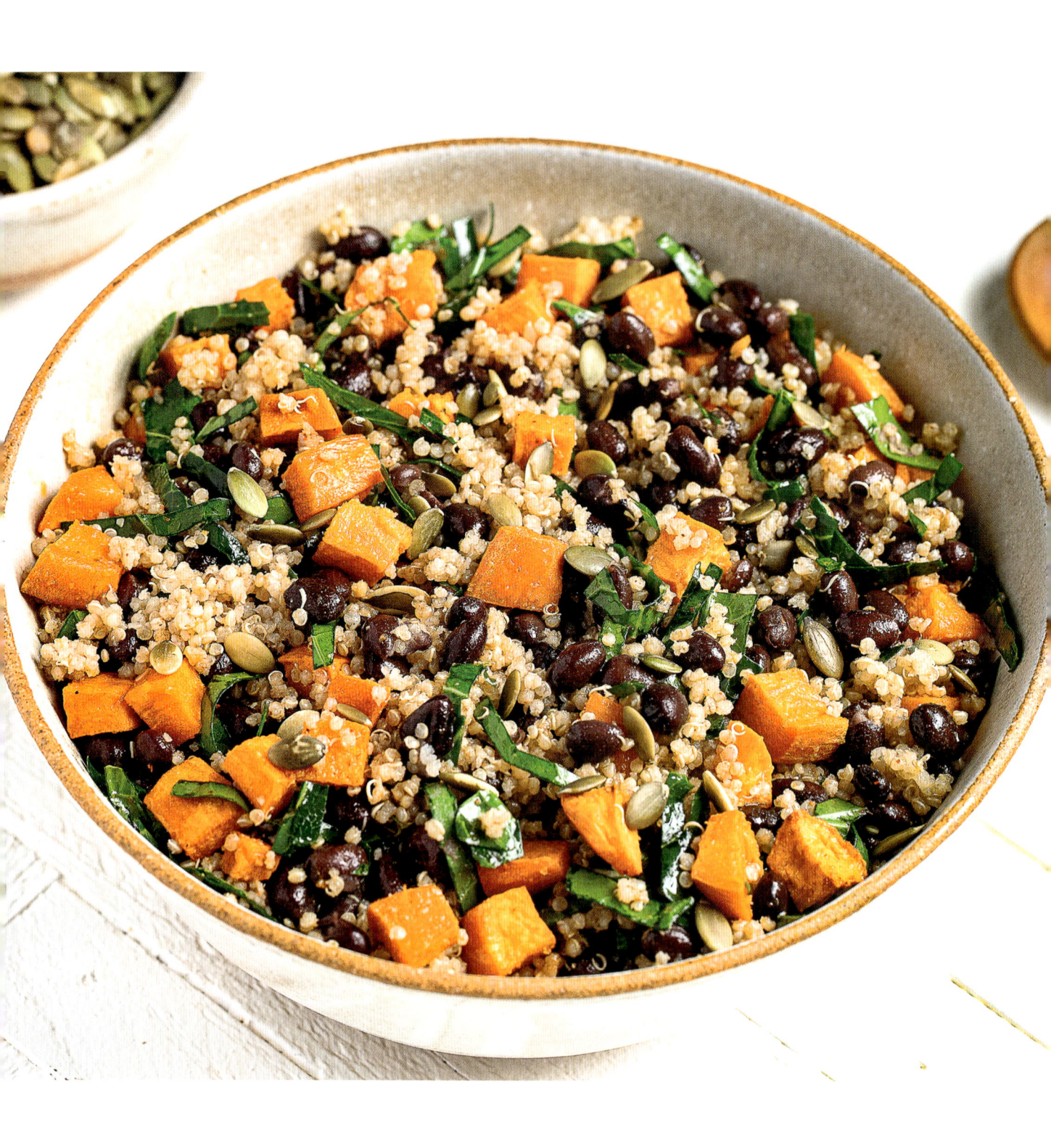

ROASTED SWEET POTATO, QUINOA & KALE SALAD

This is a delicious recipe that is very versatile. You can substitute the sweet potatoes for roasted winter squash or use pinto or garbanzo beans in place of black beans. You can also substitute the kale for any chopped greens; romaine lettuce is also a great option. If you want some extra protein, add some roasted chicken breast to this salad. The quinoa can be made the day before.

INGREDIENTS

SWEET POTATOES:

- 2 medium-sized sweet potatoes, peeled and cut into ½-inch to 1-inch cubes
- 2 tablespoons avocado oil
- ½ teaspoon garlic powder
- ½ teaspoon sea salt
- ¼ teaspoon pepper (optional; omit if nightshade-free)

DRESSING:

- ¼ cup olive oil
- 3–4 tablespoons apple cider vinegar
- 1 garlic clove, minced
- 1 teaspoon Dijon mustard
- 1 teaspoon chili powder (optional; omit if nightshade-free)
- ¾ teaspoon sea salt

SALAD:

- 2 (15-ounce) cans black beans, drained and rinsed
- 3 cups cooked quinoa
- 2–3 cups thinly sliced kale, chard, or collard leaves
- ¼–½ cup chopped cilantro (optional)
- Pumpkin seeds (optional)

INSTRUCTIONS

1. Preheat the oven to 400°F.

2. Spread sweet potatoes out on a parchment-paper-lined baking sheet and drizzle with avocado oil.

3. Sprinkle garlic powder, salt, and pepper over sweet potatoes, mix well, and spread evenly on the sheet.

4. Bake for 35–40 minutes or until soft. Remove from oven and allow them to cool while you prepare the dressing.

5. In a small bowl, whisk together the olive oil, vinegar, garlic, mustard, chili powder, and salt.

6. Place black beans, cooked quinoa, kale, cilantro, and sweet potatoes in a large bowl. Add dressing and toss well to combine.

7. Add extra salt, pepper, cilantro, or chili powder to taste.

8. Top with pumpkin seeds, if desired.

COOK TIME: 45 MINUTES
SERVES 4–6

> Sweet potatoes are not considered a nightshade, even though they have the word potato in their name. They are considered a complex carbohydrate, which helps to stabilize your blood sugar and reduce blood glucose levels. Sweet potatoes are also loaded with antioxidants that help our bodies fight against free radical damage.

ROASTED VEGETABLE & KALE SALAD WITH APPLE CIDER VINAIGRETTE

Prepare this roasted vegetable salad any time of year using any seasonal produce you have on hand. This root vegetable version is best for fall or winter; in spring or summer months, substitute vegetables like fennel, beets, zucchini, snap peas, cauliflower, or broccoli. Feel free to add any of your favorite spices; the recipe adapts well to any palate!

INGREDIENTS

- 1 medium sweet potato, cut into 1-inch cubes
- 1 medium turnip, cut into 1-inch cubes
- 2 large carrots, cut into thick rounds
- 1 medium celeriac or parsnip, peeled and cut into 1-inch pieces
- 1 medium red onion, sliced into half-moons
- 3–4 tablespoons avocado oil, divided
- 1 teaspoon dried thyme
- ¾ teaspoon sea salt
- 4 cups chopped kale (about 1 bunch)
- Pinch of sea salt

DRESSING

- 2 tablespoons apple cider vinegar
- 2 tablespoons olive oil
- 1 teaspoon Dijon mustard
- 1 teaspoon minced garlic (optional)
- ½ teaspoon sea salt

INSTRUCTIONS

1. Preheat oven to 425°F and line a large baking sheet with parchment paper.

2. Add sweet potatoes, turnips, carrots, celeriac/parsnips, and onions to baking sheet. Drizzle with 2–3 tablespoons avocado oil, sprinkle with thyme and salt, and stir to coat vegetables evenly. Spread vegetables evenly on baking sheet.

3. Bake vegetables for 30–40 minutes or until soft.

4. While vegetables are roasting, whisk all dressing ingredients in a small bowl and set aside.

5. Next, place chopped kale in a large bowl and drizzle with 1 tablespoon of avocado oil. Add a pinch of sea salt and mix well to coat.

6. When vegetables are done, remove them from oven. Add kale to pan, tucking it between roasted vegetables.

7. Transfer pan back to oven for an additional 2–3 minutes or until kale is wilted.

8. Remove pan from oven and transfer vegetables and kale to a large bowl. Drizzle dressing on top and toss well to coat.

9. Serve warm and adjust salt to taste.

COOK TIME: 45 MINUTES
SERVES 4-6

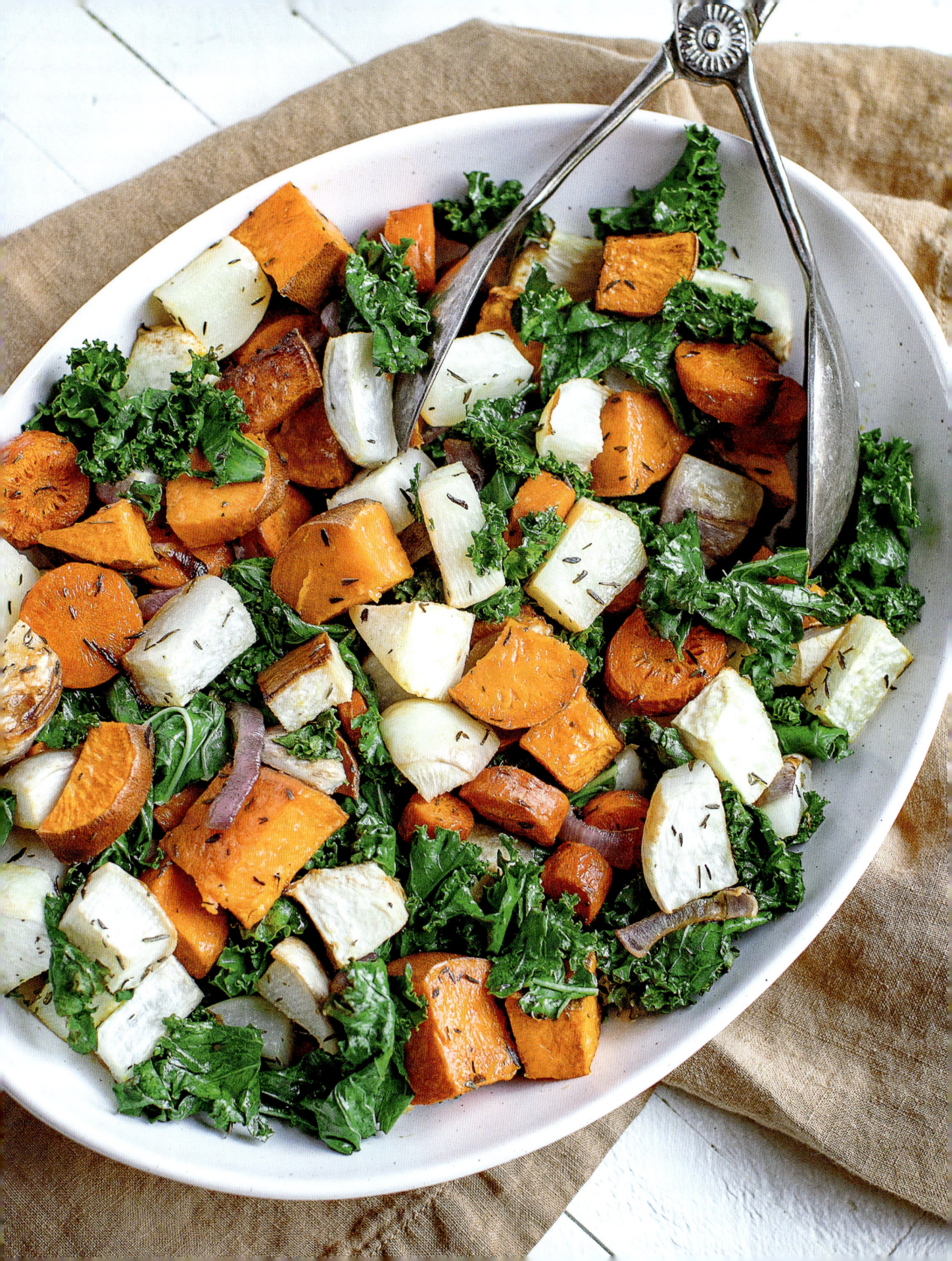

SNAP PEA, RADISH & MINT SALAD

This is a great crunchy salad to have as a snack or lunch with added protein, such as roasted chicken or salmon. Try it with extra snap peas, extra mint, or any added vegetables. Store leftover dressing in the refrigerator for up to a week.

INGREDIENTS

- 2–3 cups chopped salad mix or lettuce of choice
- 2 cups thinly sliced snap peas
- 1 cup shredded red cabbage, green cabbage, and/or carrots
- 1 cup matchstick-cut radishes
- 10 fresh mint leaves, sliced thin

DRESSING:
- ¼ cup olive oil plus 2 tablespoons
- ¼ cup apple cider vinegar (or additional lemon juice)
- 1 tablespoon lemon juice
- 2 garlic cloves, minced
- 1 teaspoon sea salt

INSTRUCTIONS

1. Add salad greens, snap peas, cabbage/carrots, radishes, and mint to a medium-sized bowl and toss well to combine.

2. Whisk together oil, vinegar, lemon juice, garlic, and salt.

3. Pour desired amount of dressing over salad and toss well.

4. Serve and garnish with extra mint if desired.

PREP TIME: 20 MINUTES
SERVES 4

> Snap peas are a sweet, crunchy, and delicious addition to any salad. They are part of the legume family and have an edible pod that is best eaten raw or slightly cooked. Not only are snap peas a great source of vitamins C and K, they also have a low glycemic index and each cup of sliced snap peas provides 2 milligrams of iron and 2 grams of protein! Snap peas contain both soluble and insoluble fiber, which promote regularity by adding bulk to the stool and moving food through the digestive tract.

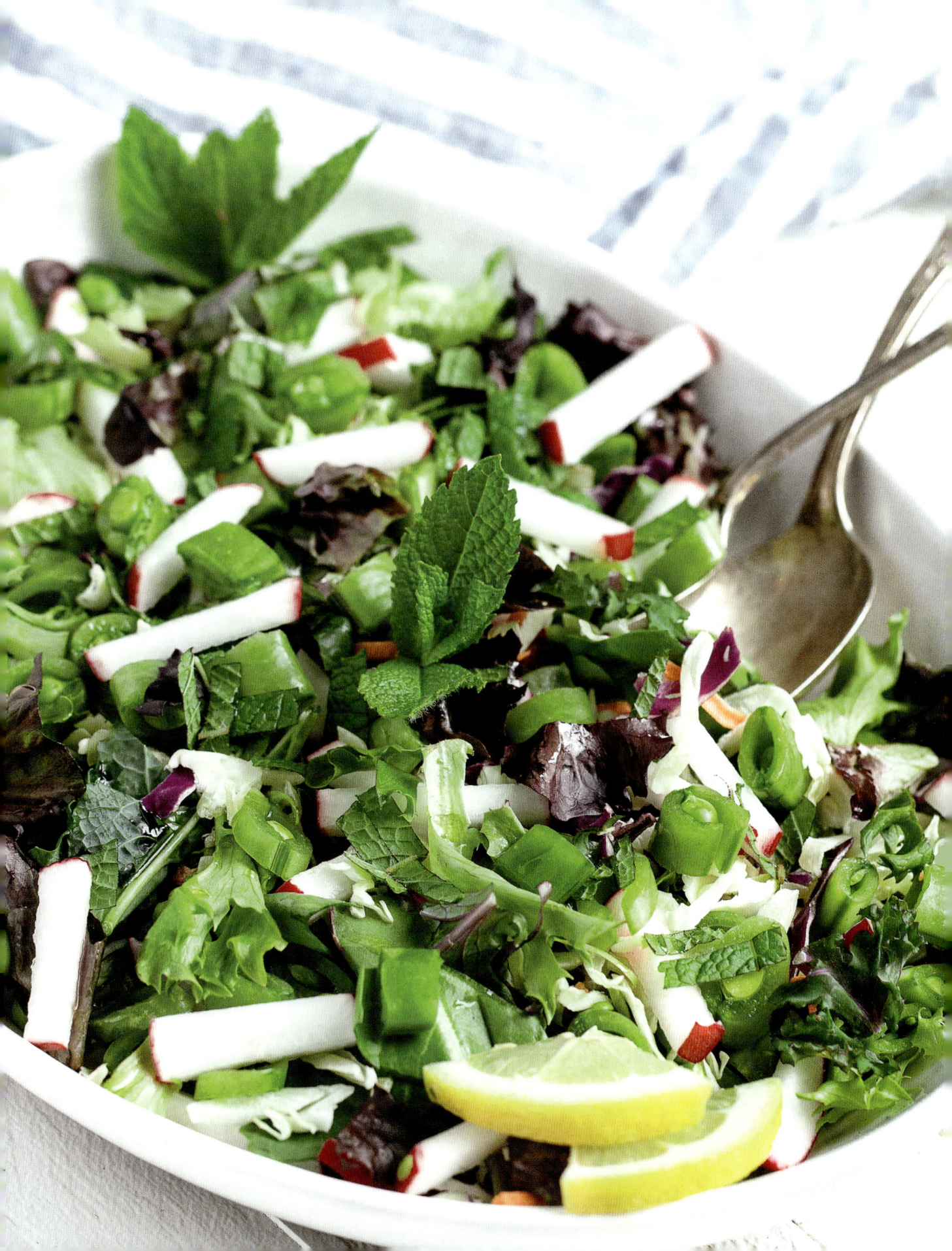

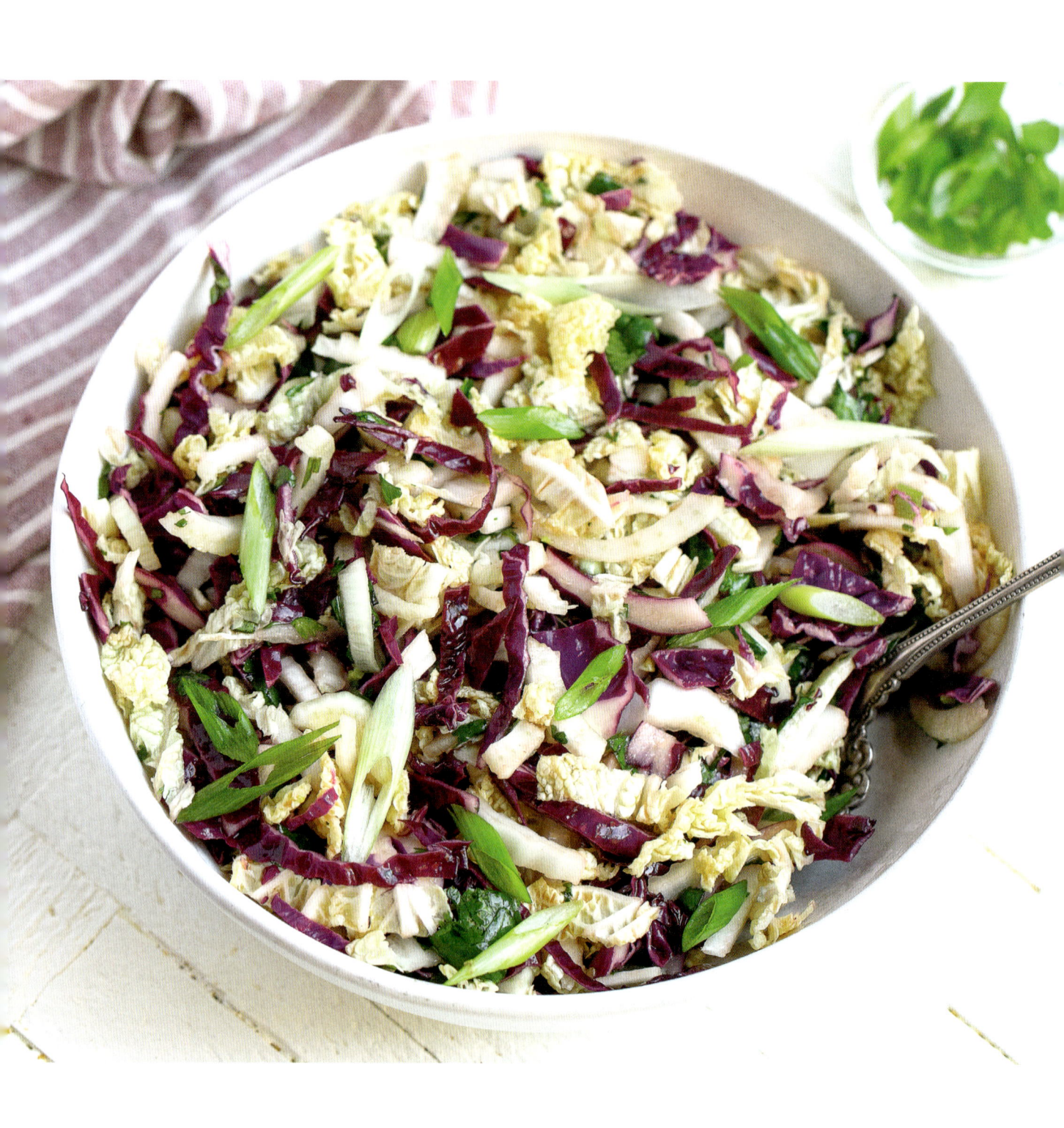

RAINBOW-CABBAGE FENNEL SLAW

Add a diverse range of vegetables to your diet with this slaw. You can include any type of cabbage or julienned vegetables. Try adding some fresh mint or a squeeze of lime for extra flavor. Store in an airtight glass container in the refrigerator for up to 4 days.

INGREDIENTS

- ½ small red cabbage, shredded
- ½ small napa or savoy cabbage, sliced thin
- 1 medium fennel bulb, sliced thin
- 2 green onions, sliced thin
- ¼ cup chopped cilantro
- ¼ cup chopped fresh basil
- ¼ cup olive oil
- 3 tablespoons apple cider vinegar
- 2 teaspoons coconut aminos
- ¼ teaspoon sea salt
- Chopped fresh mint (optional)
- Lime juice (optional)

INSTRUCTIONS

1. Add red cabbage, green cabbage, fennel, green onions, cilantro, and basil to a medium-sized bowl.

2. In a separate small bowl, whisk oil, vinegar, coconut aminos, and salt together.

3. Drizzle dressing over vegetables and toss well to combine. Add additional salt to taste.

4. Top with extra cilantro, sliced green onions, chopped fresh mint, or a squeeze of lime if desired.

PREP TIME: 10 MINUTES
SERVES 4-5

WILD SALMON SALAD

The fresh baked wild salmon in this salad is a great source of omega-3s, which have a variety of benefits. It stores well in the refrigerator and is a great option for a quick lunch. It's delicious wrapped in a coconut tortilla, lettuce, or collard leaf.

INGREDIENTS

BAKED SALMON
1 (1½-pound) wild-caught salmon fillet
2 teaspoons olive or avocado oil
¼ teaspoon sea salt
Juice of ½ small lemon or ¼ large lemon

SALAD
3 celery ribs, chopped
1 green onion, white & green parts sliced thin
2 tablespoons fresh dill, or 2 teaspoons dried
Juice of ½ lemon or more to taste
¼–½ teaspoon sea salt
2 tablespoons avocado oil
Pinch of pepper

INSTRUCTIONS

1. Preheat oven to 400°F.

2. Place salmon in a 9×13-inch glass baking dish.

3. Drizzle with oil and sprinkle with salt, pepper, and a squeeze of lemon.

4. Bake for 20 minutes or until cooked through.

5. Remove from oven and allow to cool completely while preparing other ingredients.

6. In a large bowl, add celery, green onion, dill, lemon juice, sea salt, and cooled salmon with skin removed and mix well.

7. Add the avocado oil and mix ingredients together to coat well. Add additional salt and/or lemon to taste.

8. Serve or store in refrigerator for 3–4 days.

COOK TIME: 30 MINUTES
SERVES 3–4

> Salmon is a cold-water fish that is best consumed from wild-caught sources. Not only is salmon a great source of clean protein, it's also a good source of omega-3 fatty acids. One of the things that makes processed foods so unhealthy is the use of omega-6 oils, like sunflower oil and safflower oil, which create an imbalance in the ratio of omega-3s to omega-6s. We want more omega-3s, so eating wild-caught salmon a few times a week is a great way to keep that ratio in check.

APPLE, NUT BUTTER & CHIA BOATS

A great snack for when you feel like your blood sugar is low and needs some support ASAP! You can use any fruits you have on hand; this combination of ingredients is especially good with sliced pears, apples, or bananas.

INGREDIENTS

2–3 apples
¼ cup nut butter of choice
3 tablespoons chia seeds
½–1 teaspoon cinnamon
3 tablespoons finely shredded coconut (optional)

INSTRUCTIONS

1. Cut apples into ¼-inch slices and spread out on a plate.

2. Spread 1–2 teaspoons of nut butter on top of each slice.

3. Sprinkle chia seeds on top of all apples and finish each with a dash of cinnamon and shredded coconut if desired.

PREP TIME: 5 MINUTES

SERVES 2–3

EVERYTHING ALMOND FLOUR CRACKERS

These crackers are a great high-protein snack and also incredibly easy to make. Adjust the salt in the batter according to the seasoning mix you use (use less salt if the mix is salted).

INGREDIENTS

1½ cups almond flour
2 tablespoons chia seeds
1 tablespoon ground flaxseeds
1 tablespoon Everything But The Bagel seasoning or any other dried herb seasoning
¼–½ teaspoon sea salt
3 tablespoons water, plus more as needed
2 tablespoons avocado oil

INSTRUCTIONS

1. Preheat oven to 325°F.

2. Mix all dry ingredients together in a bowl and break up any clumps. Slowly add water and oil, mixing well with a wooden spoon. You may need to add a little more water to help the dough form.

3. Use your hands to form the dough into a ball.

4. Place a sheet of parchment paper on a large cutting board and put the dough ball on the sheet of parchment. Add a second piece of parchment paper on top and use a rolling pin to roll dough into a ¼-inch-thick square, which should almost fit the width of a baking sheet.

5. Remove top sheet of parchment paper and transfer bottom sheet with rolled-out dough onto a baking sheet.

6. Using a pizza cutter, score crackers into desired sizes.

7. Bake for 15–18 minutes or until crackers start to brown.

8. Remove from oven. When completely cool, break into crackers.

9. Store in an airtight glass container for up to a week.

COOK TIME: 30 MINUTES

MAKES APPROXIMATELY 20 CRACKERS

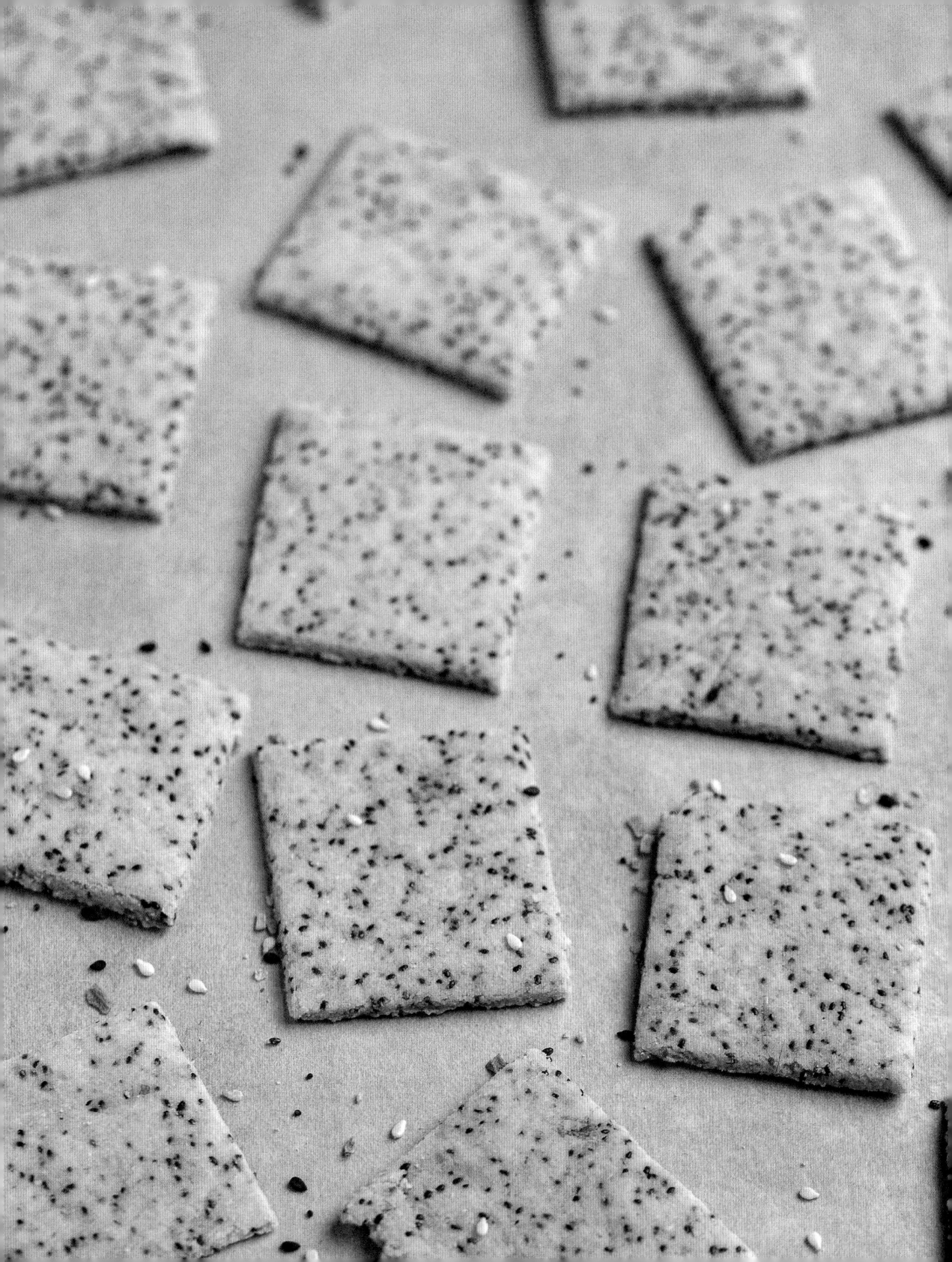

CURRY SPICED NUTS

This is a very versatile recipe that you can make on a weekly basis for a quick available snack. Pecans and cashews work well with these spices. Try mixing the two or experimenting with some of your favorite raw nuts.

INGREDIENTS

½ teaspoon curry powder

½ teaspoon sea salt

¼ teaspoon garlic powder

¼ teaspoon turmeric powder

1 tablespoon avocado oil

2 cups raw unsalted nuts (cashews, pecans, or mixed nuts)

1½ teaspoons coconut aminos

OPTIONAL

¼ teaspoon ground cinnamon

¼ teaspoon dried ground ginger

INSTRUCTIONS

1. Preheat oven to 325°F and line a baking sheet with parchment paper.

2. Add all the spices to a medium-sized mixing bowl and whisk to combine. Add nuts and oil and mix well, making sure that all nuts are evenly coated.

3. Spread nut mixture out evenly on parchment-lined baking sheet.

4. Bake for 6–8 minutes, stir, and bake for another 6–7 minutes.

5. Remove from oven and let cool.

6. Store in an airtight glass container for up to a week.

COOK TIME: 20 MINUTES

SERVES 4–6

EASY OVEN-BAKED KALE CHIPS

These kale chips are super easy and quick to make! Make sure the kale is very dry prior to adding oil and spices. You can add any spices you'd like; our favorites are curry powder and garlic. Try onion powder, Italian seasonings, or a combination of your choice.

INGREDIENTS

1 large bunch of kale (lacinato or green curly kale)
1 tablespoon avocado oil
1 teaspoon finely ground sea salt
¼ teaspoon curry powder (optional)
¼ teaspoon garlic powder (optional)

INSTRUCTIONS

1. Preheat oven to 300°F and line a large baking sheet with parchment paper.

2. Remove kale leaves from stem and discard stem. Tear leaves into large pieces and add to a mixing bowl.

3. Add avocado oil, sea salt, and any spices you might like. Toss well so that all the leaves are coated well.

4. Spread evenly on the baking sheet and bake for 20–25 minutes or until kale edges crisp up and start to brown.

5. Once cooled, store in an airtight glass container for up to 4 days.

COOK TIME: 25 MINUTES
SERVES 4–5

> Kale is a highly nutritious superfood that's known for several health benefits, including its capacity for fighting inflammation, high content of antioxidants, and plant-based omega-3 fatty acids, which help regulate the inflammatory process in the body. Kale contains high levels of vitamin C and beta-carotene that aid the body's detoxification process.

CREAMY DAIRY-FREE SPINACH-ARTICHOKE DIP

Best served warm immediately after cooking, this dip makes a great midday snack. Serve with grain-free chips, almond crackers, or cut vegetables. It also stores well for up to 4 days in the refrigerator.

INGREDIENTS

- 1 cup raw unsalted cashews
- 1 cup water
- 1 tablespoon avocado oil
- ½ medium onion, chopped
- 2 garlic cloves, minced
- 1 (14-ounce) can artichoke hearts, strained and chopped
- ½ teaspoon garlic powder
- 1 (10-ounce) box frozen spinach, thawed and chopped (squeeze out water before chopping)
- 1 (8-ounce) can water chestnuts, strained and chopped
- Juice of ½ lemon
- ½ teaspoon sea salt
- ¼ teaspoon pepper (optional; omit if nightshade-free)

INSTRUCTIONS

1. Soak cashews in 1 cup of hot water for 30 minutes. Strain and rinse, then add to a high-speed blender with 1 cup water. Blend until smooth.

2. While cashews soak, heat a medium-sized saucepan or cast-iron skillet on medium heat and add avocado oil. When hot, add onions and a pinch of salt. Cook until soft, then quickly stir in minced garlic for 15 seconds.

3. Add artichoke hearts, spinach, and water chestnuts. Cook until hot.

4. Add blended cashew mixture, lemon juice, garlic powder, and salt. Stir well. Add pepper if desired.

5. Serve warm with almond crackers or vegetables.

COOK TIME: 40 MINUTES
SERVES 4

> A major noteworthy benefit of artichokes is that they are a rich source of soluble fiber, which is important for any anti-inflammatory protocol—especially for those dealing with blood sugar issues. An anti-inflammatory powerhouse, the artichoke is considered one of the most antioxidant-rich vegetables you can eat.

EASY CHICKPEA SOCCA

One of the hardest things to give up on an anti-inflammatory diet is bread. This chickpea socca can serve as a substitute when you are craving bread and can be used as a base for any type of sandwich, eaten with avocado on top, or served simply as is. It is best straight out of the oven, but it can be stored at room temperature for a day and reheated at 400°F until the edges crisp up again.

INGREDIENTS

1 cup chickpea flour
1 cup water
3 tablespoons olive or avocado oil, divided
½ teaspoon sea salt
½ teaspoon garlic powder (optional)

INSTRUCTIONS

1. In a medium bowl, combine chickpea flour, water, 2 tablespoons oil, salt, and garlic powder. Whisk until very smooth, making sure to whisk out any lumps. Set aside and allow to thicken for 30 minutes.

2. Preheat oven to 475°F with a 10-inch cast-iron skillet inside.

3. Using a pot holder, remove preheated skillet from oven and add remaining 1 tablespoon oil, swirling to coat the bottom and sides of the pan. Pour batter into the hot pan and bake for 18–20 minutes or until socca looks brown and crisp around the edges. You can turn the heat up to broil for a minute or two if you want to crisp the top, but keep an eye on it so it doesn't burn.

4. Remove from the oven, let cool slightly, and then slice into quarters. Use a spatula to transfer socca from the skillet to a serving plate.

5. Enjoy as is or top it with spices, avocado, dips, or dressings!

COOK TIME: 50 MINUTES
SERVES 2–3

MAIN DISHES

Instead of using processed foods, which make up some of the most common food intolerances, these recipes feature healthy and lean sources of protein and plenty of nutrient-dense vegetables. Each main dish will reduce inflammation in your body while at the same time giving it the many nutrients it needs to function optimally.

What and when you eat make a huge difference in how your body functions and how you feel. During your Inflammatory Reset, aim to make lunch your largest meal of the day. While keeping this in mind, always eat according to your appetite and don't overeat! The trick is to slow down—and even enjoy—your midday meal instead of rushing to the next task as many of us do. For dinner, try to eat earlier in the evening because your metabolism slows as the daylight hours fade. A smaller dinner works best with the Inflammatory Reset. These main dishes will ensure you get plenty of vegetables and proteins in every meal to create some balance and energy for your day.

- Vegetable Stir-Fry
- Chicken Tacos in Cabbage Leaf Wraps
- Ground Lamb Taco Bowl with Creamy Cilantro Dressing
- Curried Lentil, Cauliflower & Kale Bowl
- Crispy Salmon, Sweet Potato & Quinoa Bowl with Carrot-Ginger Dressing
- Sheet-Pan Chicken with Cauliflower, Carrots & Greens
- One-Pan Roasted Salmon & Vegetables
- Salmon Quinoa Cakes
- Quick Asian Turkey Wraps
- Lentil Pasta with Garlicky Roasted Cauliflower
- Sheet-Pan Fish & Vegetable Fajitas
- Shepherd's Pie with Cauliflower Crust
- Whole Roasted Chicken with Vegetables

VEGETABLE STIR-FRY

This stir-fry is very easy to throw together for a quick lunch or dinner. If you like ginger, add more for a spicier stir-fry. Serve on top of a bed of quinoa or millet, or serve as is for a complete meal.

INGREDIENTS

- 1 pound boneless, skinless chicken breast, cut into bite-sized pieces
- ¼ teaspoon sea salt
- Dash of pepper (optional; omit if nightshade-free)
- 3 tablespoons avocado oil, divided
- 1 medium shallot, chopped
- 2 carrots, peeled and cut into matchsticks
- 3 cups broccoli florets
- 1 zucchini, cut into ¼-inch cubes
- 3 tablespoons coconut aminos
- 1 tablespoon grated fresh ginger

INSTRUCTIONS

1. Place chicken in a bowl and toss with salt and pepper to coat evenly.

2. Heat 1 tablespoon avocado oil in a large skillet on medium-high heat. Once hot, add chicken in a single layer, careful not to overcrowd the pan. Work in batches if necessary.

3. Sear chicken on both sides for 5–7 minutes, tossing occasionally until cooked through so pieces are not pink and are browned on the edges. Transfer to a plate.

4. Add remaining 2 tablespoons oil to pan, then add shallots, carrots, broccoli, and zucchini.

5. Cook for 4–5 minutes, stirring occasionally, until vegetables are slightly tender.

6. Return chicken to pan along with ginger and coconut aminos. Stir all ingredients together until chicken is hot. Turn off heat and add more salt or coconut aminos to taste if desired.

7. Serve as is or on top of a bed of quinoa or millet.

COOK TIME: 30 MINUTES
SERVES 4

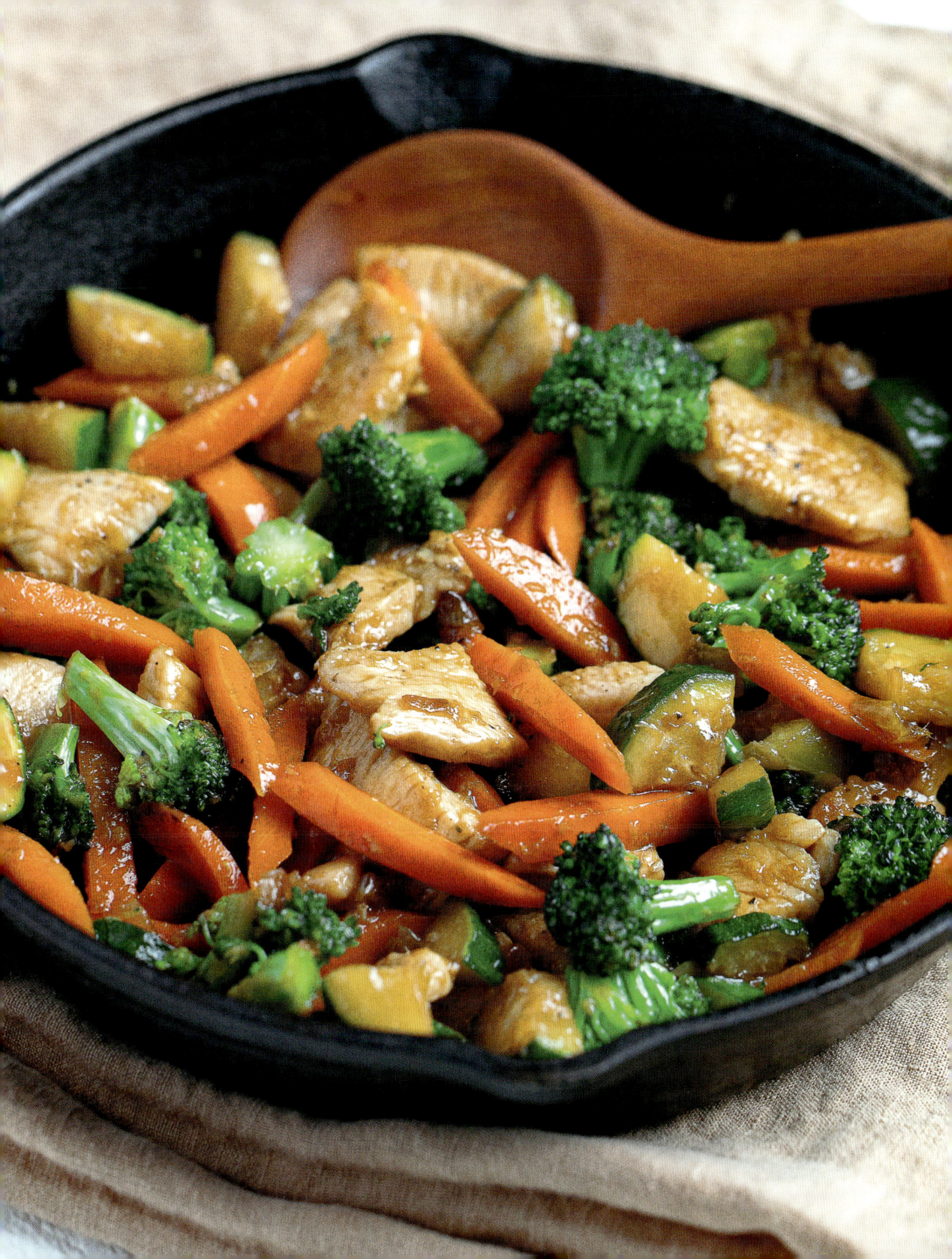

CHICKEN TACOS IN CABBAGE LEAF WRAPS

Packed with flavor and healthy fats, these tacos are a delicious alternative to traditional tacos. Add any chopped vegetables, more avocado, or hot sauce to create your own version to suit your taste.

INGREDIENTS

2 medium boneless, skinless chicken breasts

1 teaspoon sea salt

¼–½ teaspoon garlic powder

Pinch of black pepper (optional; omit if nightshade-free)

2 tablespoons avocado or coconut oil

1 avocado, cubed

6 red or green cabbage leaves, cut into taco-shell shapes

1 red bell pepper, chopped (optional; omit if nightshade-free)

6 red radishes, sliced into matchsticks

¼ cup chopped cilantro

Dash of hot sauce (optional)

1 lime, cut into wedges

INSTRUCTIONS

1. Season chicken breasts generously with salt, garlic powder, and pepper.

2. Heat oil in a large skillet on medium heat.

3. Add chicken to the heated pan and cover partially with a lid.

4. Cook for 3–5 minutes or until chicken begins to brown and tops begin to turn white. Flip and cook for another 3–5 minutes or until cooked through and the internal temperature is 165°F.

5. Remove chicken from pan and let cool for 5–7 minutes. When cool, cut chicken into small cubes.

6. Arrange cabbage leaf "shells" on a plate and add chicken, bell pepper, avocado, radish, and cilantro to the shells.

7. Serve with hot sauce and a squeeze of lime on top of each taco if desired.

COOK TIME: 20 MINUTES
SERVES 6

GROUND LAMB TACO BOWL WITH CREAMY CILANTRO DRESSING

This recipe is very adaptable. Use ground turkey or chicken instead of lamb, add any vegetables, omit the dressing, or add extra hot sauce to change it up. Store leftovers in the refrigerator in an airtight glass container for up to 3 days.

INGREDIENTS

DRESSING
- 1 cup hemp seeds
- ¾ cup olive oil
- ¾ cup water
- ¼ cup lemon juice
- 2 tablespoons coconut aminos
- 1 garlic clove, minced
- ¾ teaspoon sea salt
- 1 cup packed cilantro leaves

GROUND LAMB
- 1 pound grass-fed ground lamb
- 2 tablespoons coconut aminos
- 2 teaspoons chili powder (optional; omit if nightshade-free)
- ½ teaspoon sea salt
- ½ teaspoon garlic powder
- ½ teaspoon ground cumin
- ½ teaspoon dried oregano

OPTIONAL
- Romaine lettuce
- Shredded red or green cabbage
- Sliced radishes
- Chopped cilantro
- Sliced red peppers (omit if nightshade-free)
- Shredded carrots
- Sliced avocado
- Cooked quinoa
- Leftover roasted vegetables
- Any other vegetables, nuts, or seeds of choice

INSTRUCTIONS

1. For dressing, add hemp seeds, olive oil, water, lemon juice, coconut aminos, garlic, and sea salt to a blender and blend until smooth. Then add cilantro leaves and blend briefly until dressing turns green. Add additional salt to taste.

2. Heat a large skillet on medium-high heat. Crumble lamb into skillet and cook until browned, 7–10 minutes. Drain excess grease from pan, return to heat, and lower to medium.

3. Add all seasonings and cook for an additional 8–10 minutes or until all seasonings are absorbed and meat is cooked through. Taste, adding extra salt and pepper if desired.

4. Assemble taco bowls by adding lamb, optional ingredients, dressing, hot sauce if desired, and any other toppings.

COOK TIME: 25 MINUTES
SERVES 3–4

> Lamb in moderation is a health-promoting source of protein that is rich in selenium, zinc, and iron. Though lamb is considered a red meat, the protein and minerals your body absorbs from eating it make it okay to include in the Inflammatory Reset.

CURRIED LENTIL, CAULIFLOWER & KALE BOWL

This is a recipe that you can keep in the refrigerator and heat as needed. All components can be reheated individually or together as a bowl with your favorite vegetables, quinoa, or millet added. Garnish with chopped fresh herbs like cilantro or green onions before serving.

INGREDIENTS

CAULIFLOWER & KALE
1 medium cauliflower, cut into florets
3 tablespoons avocado oil, divided
½–1 teaspoon garlic powder
½ teaspoon sea salt
3–4 cups chopped green kale

LENTILS
6 cups water
2 cups red lentils, rinsed
2 tablespoons avocado oil
1 medium shallot, chopped
2 garlic cloves, minced
2 tablespoons fresh ginger, minced
2 tablespoons Madras curry powder
½ teaspoon sea salt
1 (13.5-ounce) can coconut milk
2 tablespoons coconut aminos
¼ cup lemon juice, plus more to taste
Cooked quinoa or millet (optional)
Garnish of chopped cilantro or green onions

INSTRUCTIONS

CAULIFLOWER & KALE INSTRUCTIONS

1. Preheat oven to 400°F and line a baking sheet with parchment paper.

2. Spread cauliflower florets out on pan and drizzle 2 tablespoons avocado oil on top.

3. Sprinkle garlic powder and sea salt over cauliflower. Toss well to coat and spread out on pan evenly.

4. Bake for 30 minutes or until florets start to brown.

5. Remove pan from oven and push cauliflower to one side. Add kale, remaining 1 tablespoon oil, and a large pinch of sea salt to the other side.

6. Toss kale well and spread out on the empty half of the pan.

7. Return pan to oven for 5 minutes or until kale is wilted and bright green.

8. Remove from oven and let cool before assembling your bowl.

LENTILS INSTRUCTIONS

1. Add water and a large pinch of salt to a medium pot and bring to a boil. Add lentils and reduce heat to a simmer. Cook uncovered for 15–18 minutes or until lentils are cooked through. Strain off any excess water and set aside.

2. Heat oil in a skillet on medium heat.

3. Add shallots and a pinch of salt and cook until soft. Add minced garlic and cook for an additional minute until fragrant.

4. Add ginger, curry powder, and salt and cook for 1 minute. Add coconut milk and coconut aminos.

5. Bring to a boil. Simmer for 5–10 minutes, then add cooked lentils and stir well.

6. Turn off heat and add lemon juice. Add extra salt or lemon juice to taste.

7. Create your bowl by adding cooked quinoa or millet if desired, curried lentils, cauliflower, and kale. Top with fresh chopped cilantro and/or green onions.

COOK TIME: 45 MINUTES
SERVES 6

> Part of the legume family, lentils have been known to help lower blood pressure and cholesterol. They are high in protein, vitamin B6, magnesium, calcium, and vitamin C. Lentils contain high amounts of polyphenols, which help reduce inflammation, improve heart health, and boost brain function.

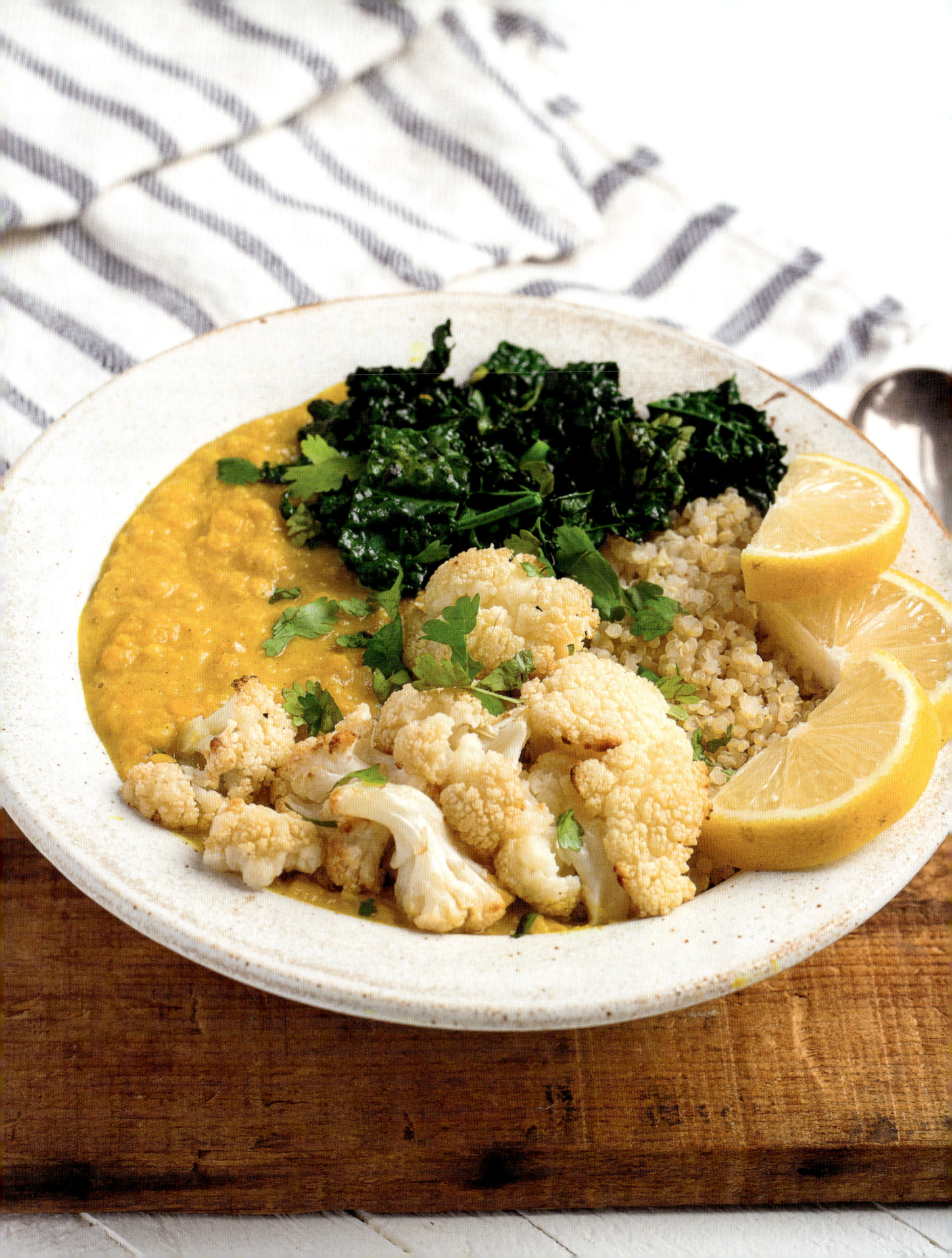

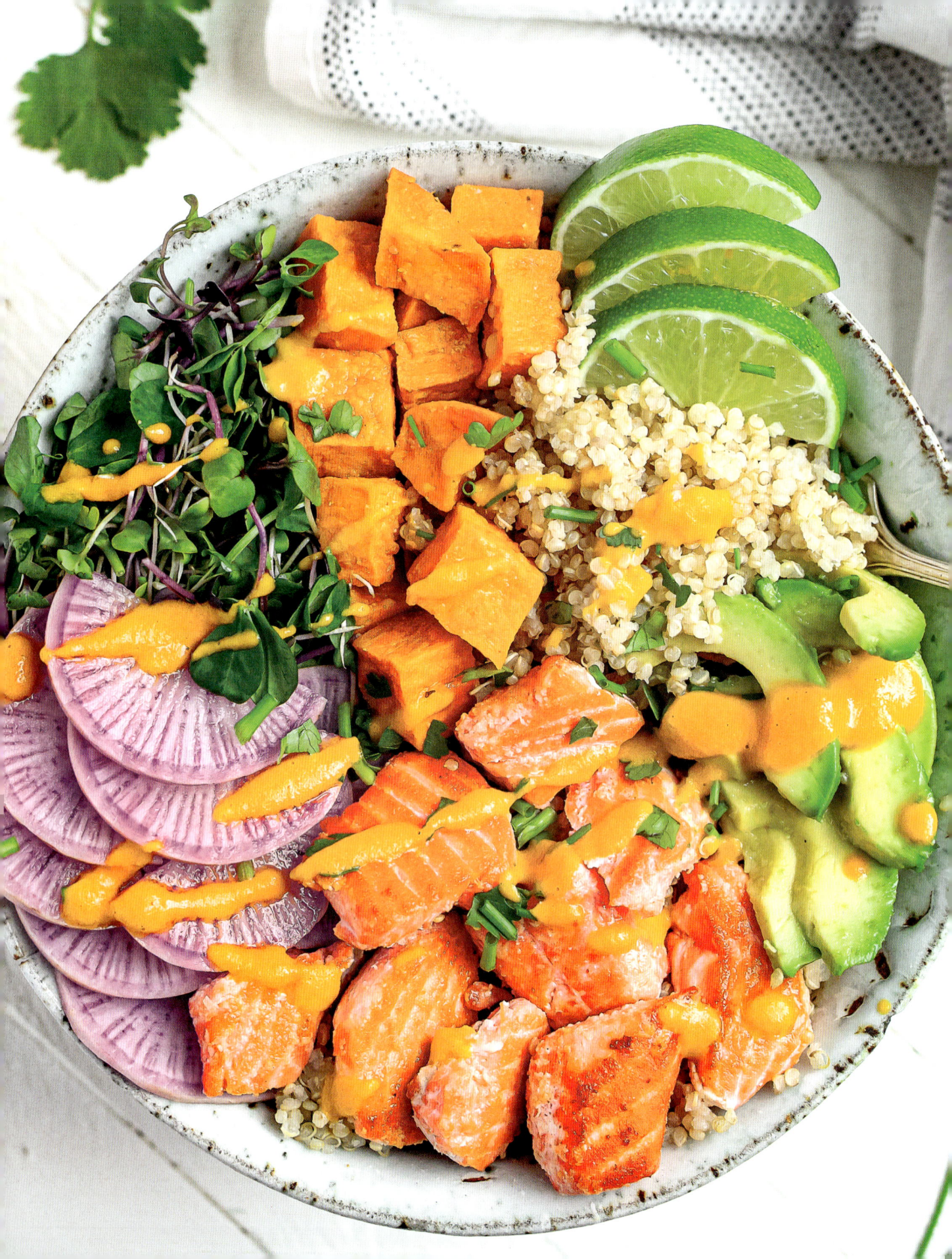

CRISPY SALMON, SWEET POTATO & QUINOA BOWL WITH CARROT-GINGER DRESSING

This bowl is very adaptable. Omit any ingredients you are sensitive to and substitute whatever you'd like! Add any raw or roasted vegetables that are in season or that you're craving. All ingredients can be made ahead of time and stored in the refrigerator for a quick lunch.

INGREDIENTS

3–4 cups quinoa

1 large or 2 medium-sized sweet potatoes, peeled and cut into ½- or 1-inch cubes

2 tablespoons avocado oil

½ teaspoon garlic powder

½ teaspoon sea salt

DRESSING

⅓ cup plus ¼ cup olive oil

¼ cup apple cider vinegar

¼ cup coconut aminos

2 medium carrots, peeled and grated

1 tablespoon peeled and finely grated fresh ginger

1 tablespoon lime juice

Pinch of sea salt

SALMON

1 pound wild-caught salmon, skin removed, cut into 1½-inch cubes

¼ teaspoon garlic powder

¼ teaspoon onion powder

¼ teaspoon sea salt

2 tablespoons avocado oil

OPTIONAL BOWL INGREDIENTS

Avocado

Chives

Cilantro

Basil

Cucumber

Radish

Sprouts

INSTRUCTIONS

1. Preheat oven to 400°F. Line a baking sheet with parchment paper.

2. Cook quinoa (according to package instructions) and set aside to cool. Quinoa can also be made the day before.

3. Spread sweet potatoes out on baking sheet and drizzle with oil.

4. Sprinkle garlic powder and sea salt over sweet potatoes. Mix well and rearrange them evenly on the sheet.

5. Bake for 35–40 minutes or until soft. Remove from oven and let cool.

6. While sweet potatoes are roasting, prepare the dressing by adding ⅓ cup olive oil, apple cider vinegar, coconut aminos, carrots, ginger, lime juice, and salt to a blender and blend well. Add additional ¼ cup olive oil and slowly blend until completely smooth. Transfer to a glass jar and set aside.

7. Next, add salmon, garlic powder, onion powder, and salt to a bowl and toss well.

8. Add avocado oil to a medium-sized skillet and heat on medium to medium-high heat until hot. Add salmon pieces and cook 3–4 minutes per side, gently turning until cooked through. Transfer salmon to a paper-towel-lined plate while preparing bowls.

9. Add quinoa, salmon, and any desired optional ingredients to a bowl, drizzle with carrot-ginger dressing, and serve.

COOK TIME: 40 MINUTES
SERVES 2–3

The carrots in this dressing are what give this dish an extra nutrient-dense boost. Carrots are loaded with fiber, which helps support the gastrointestinal tract, and packed with the antioxidant beta-carotene. Eating more orange vegetables has been associated with a decreased risk of cardiovascular disease by lowering the body's burden that is caused by oxidative stress.

SHEET-PAN CHICKEN WITH CAULIFLOWER, CARROTS & GREENS

This recipe is an easy full meal to make when you are short on time. Great for a weeknight, it pairs well with a side of quinoa or a fresh salad. You can add different vegetables to the mix, such as broccoli or any root vegetables. If you prefer white meat, substitute small split chicken breasts for the thighs. Garnish your chicken with fresh chopped herbs such as Italian parsley, rosemary, or thyme.

INGREDIENTS

- 1 small cauliflower, cut into 1-inch florets
- 2 medium carrots, cut into thick matchsticks
- 3 garlic cloves, minced
- 4 tablespoons avocado or olive oil, divided
- 1 tablespoon apple cider vinegar
- 2 teaspoons smoked paprika (optional; omit if nightshade-free)
- 1½ teaspoons sea salt
- 1 teaspoon dried thyme
- 2 pounds bone-in, skin-on chicken thighs
- 3–4 cups chopped lacinato or green kale
- Chopped fresh parsley, rosemary, or thyme (optional)
- 1 lemon, cut into wedges (optional)

INSTRUCTIONS

1. Preheat oven to 400°F and line a baking sheet with parchment paper.

2. In a very large bowl or glass baking dish, combine cauliflower, carrots, garlic, 3 tablespoons oil, vinegar, paprika, salt, and thyme. Toss to coat all vegetables. Add chicken to the bowl and toss well to coat everything.

3. Spread chicken and vegetables out on the parchment-lined sheet pan. Add additional oil to coat chicken pieces if needed. Sprinkle with a bit of salt and place in oven for 40 minutes.

4. While chicken and vegetables are roasting, add chopped kale to a medium bowl and toss well with remaining 1 tablespoon olive oil and a generous pinch of salt. Set aside.

5. After chicken has roasted for 40 minutes and the internal temperature is around 165°F–170°F, remove pan from oven. Push chicken and vegetables to one side of the pan to make room for kale.

6. Add kale to the other side of the pan, then return to the oven for 5 minutes or until kale is wilted.

7. Remove pan from oven and move chicken to one side of the sheet pan. Stir vegetables and kale together. Combine well.

8. Before serving, garnish with chopped fresh parsley, thyme, or rosemary and lemon wedges if desired.

COOK TIME: 1 HOUR
SERVES 3-4

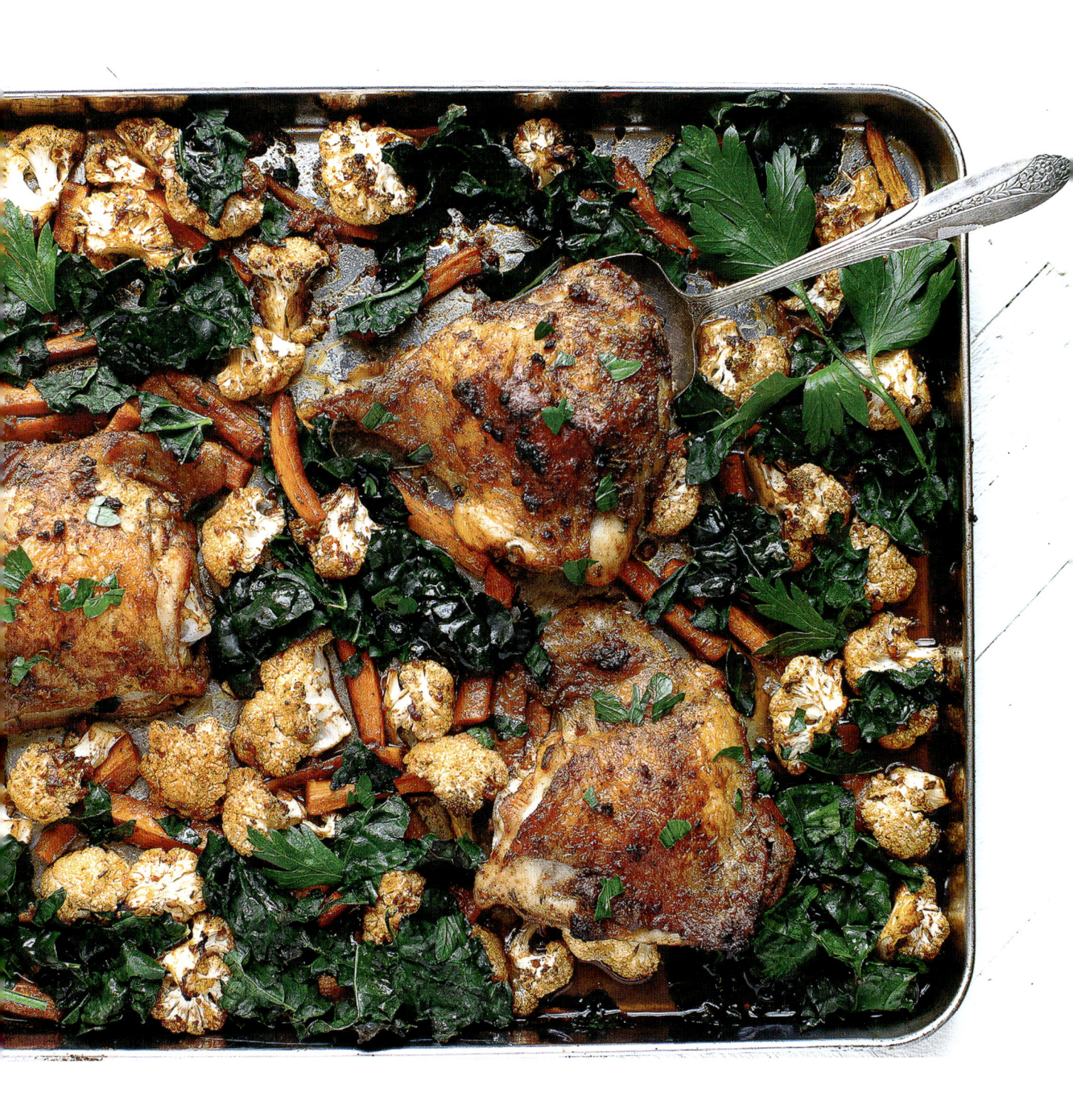

ONE-PAN ROASTED SALMON & VEGETABLES

A one-pan meal is so easy to throw together for dinner during a busy week. Switch up the vegetables according to the season: try cubed winter squash, turnips, or beets in the fall or winter, and zucchini, green beans, or snap peas during the spring or summer.

INGREDIENTS

- ½ red onion, sliced, or 1 large leek, white part sliced thin
- 3 garlic cloves, minced
- 2 cups broccoli florets
- 2 carrots, sliced
- 2 tablespoons avocado oil
- 2 tablespoons lemon juice, divided
- ¾ teaspoon sea salt, divided
- Black pepper (omit if nightshade-free)
- ¼ cup olive oil
- 3 tablespoons apple cider vinegar
- 1 tablespoon lemon juice
- ½ teaspoon Dijon mustard
- ½ teaspoon dried oregano
- 1½–2 pounds wild-caught salmon fillets
- ¼ cup chopped fresh Italian or curly parsley (optional)

INSTRUCTIONS

1. Preheat oven to 400°F.

2. Add red onion or leeks, garlic, broccoli, carrots, avocado oil, 1 tablespoon lemon juice, ½ teaspoon salt, and pepper to a medium bowl and toss well.

3. Spread vegetables out on a baking sheet lined with parchment paper and place in oven. Roast for 15 minutes.

4. While vegetables are roasting, whisk olive oil, apple cider vinegar, remaining 1 tablespoon lemon juice, mustard, oregano, remaining ¼ teaspoon salt, and pepper together in a small bowl.

5. Remove vegetables from oven and toss well. Spread them out again on the lined baking sheet.

6. Make space among vegetables and place salmon fillets on pan. Drizzle 2–3 tablespoons of dressing on top of salmon.

7. Place pan back in oven and bake for an additional 15–20 minutes or until salmon is cooked through.

8. Drizzle desired amount of extra dressing on top of salmon and vegetables. Serve topped with chopped fresh parsley.

COOK TIME: 45 MINUTES
SERVES 4–5

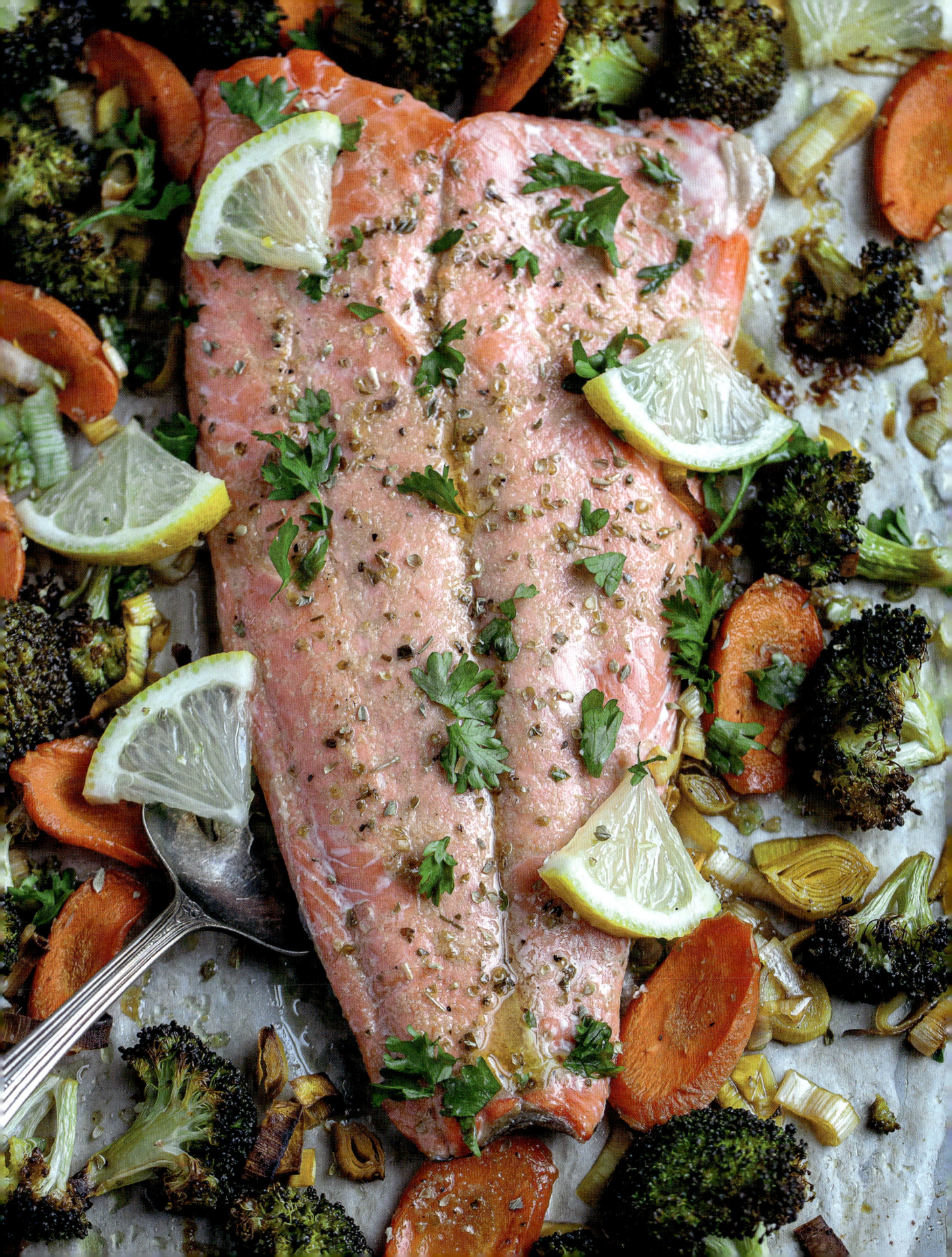

SALMON QUINOA CAKES

These salmon cakes are delicious and very easy to make. They can be served on a salad, wrapped in a lettuce or collard leaf, or served alone with a side vegetable.

INGREDIENTS

1-pound wild-caught salmon, skinned and deboned
1 teaspoon lemon zest
¾ teaspoon sea salt
½ teaspoon garlic powder
Fresh herbs, such as cilantro or parsley (optional)
1 cup cooked and cooled quinoa
2 tablespoons avocado oil

INSTRUCTIONS

1. Cut salmon into large pieces.

2. Using a food processor with an S-blade, gently pulse salmon, lemon zest, salt, and garlic powder until mixed, but not ground. If you are using fresh herbs, pulse them in now.

3. Add quinoa and pulse until all ingredients are well combined.

4. Heat a large fry pan on medium heat and add avocado oil. Once hot, add ¼ cup salmon mixture to pan at a time and flatten into ¼-inch patties.

5. Cook for 3–4 minutes or until they start to brown. Flip and cook other side until browned, an additional 1–3 minutes.

6. Remove from pan and place on a paper-towel-lined-plate to absorb oil.

7. Serve warm.

COOK TIME: 30 MINUTES
SERVES 4

QUICK ASIAN TURKEY WRAPS

This savory ground-turkey dish makes a delicious quick meal. You can substitute ground chicken for turkey, bamboo shoots for water chestnuts, and omit the red pepper if you are nightshade-free. Serve in lettuce-leaf wraps with extra cilantro, chopped red pepper, radishes, green onions, and a squeeze of lime.

INGREDIENTS

- 1 pound ground turkey (white meat, dark meat, or a combination)
- ¼ cup coconut aminos
- 1 tablespoon lime juice
- 2 garlic cloves, minced
- 2 teaspoons fresh ginger, minced
- 2 green onions, white and green parts sliced
- 1 (8-ounce) can water chestnuts, strained and chopped
- ½ cup chopped cilantro
- ¼ teaspoon sea salt
- Pinch of pepper
- 3 cups chopped lettuce

OPTIONAL TOPPINGS

- Hot sauce
- Chopped fresh herbs, such as cilantro, parsley, or basil
- Chopped radishes
- Shredded carrots
- Chopped red pepper (omit if nightshade-free)

INSTRUCTIONS

1. Heat a 12-inch pan on medium heat.

2. Crumble ground turkey and add to pan. Cook for 5–7 minutes until it is cooked through, then drain any excess liquid.

3. Add coconut aminos, lime juice, garlic, and ginger. Stir to combine. Cook for 3–5 minutes or until meat starts to absorb liquid.

4. Add green onions, water chestnuts, cilantro, salt, and pepper and stir to combine. Taste and adjust flavors to your liking. Remove from heat.

5. Serve wrapped in a lettuce or cabbage leaf with toppings of choice.

COOK TIME: 30 MINUTES
SERVES 4

> Adding good organic turkey to your diet is a great way to get ample protein into your body. Turkey is a good source of the minerals zinc, selenium, and phosphorus, and it's a good source of the sleep-promoting amino acid tryptophan. Tryptophan plays a vital role in the uptake of serotonin, which is the neurotransmitter that is involved in sleep.

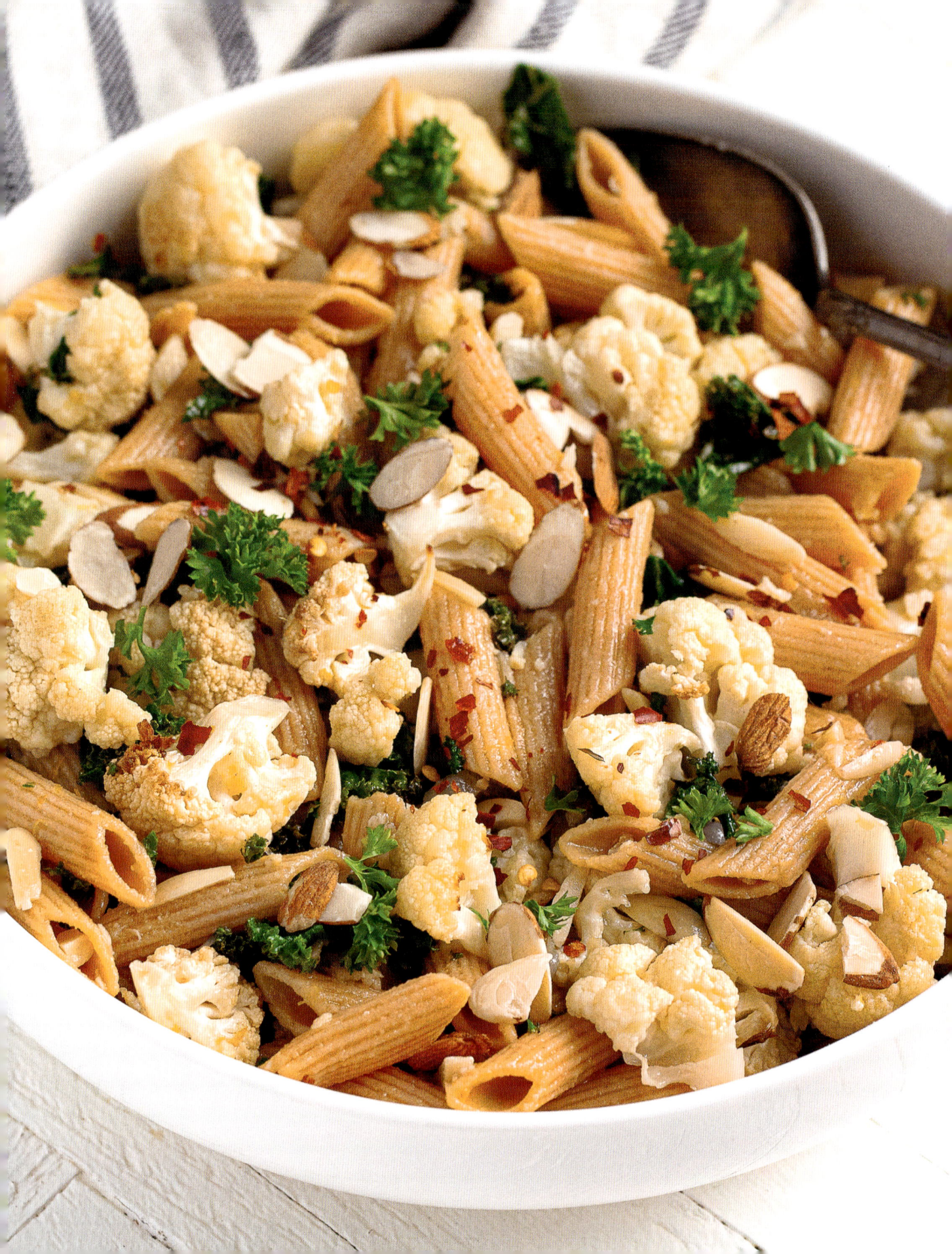

LENTIL PASTA WITH GARLICKY ROASTED CAULIFLOWER

This dish is made with lentil pasta, but you can substitute chickpea or buckwheat pasta if desired. The vegetables are easily swapped out for variety—try adding some broccoli or leeks. For some extra protein, add cubed cooked chicken breast.

INGREDIENTS

- 1 medium cauliflower, cut into bite-sized florets
- ½ medium red onion, sliced into half-moons
- 2 garlic cloves, minced
- 3 tablespoons olive or avocado oil, divided
- ½ teaspoon sea salt
- 2 cups chopped baby spinach
- 6 ounces lentil pasta, cooked and drained
- 2 teaspoons lemon zest
- ½ cup chopped fresh basil
- ¼ cup chopped walnuts or slivered almonds
- ¼ teaspoon red pepper flakes (optional; omit if nightshade-free)

INSTRUCTIONS

1. Preheat oven to 400°F.

2. Line a baking sheet with parchment paper.

3. Add cauliflower to a large bowl with red onion, garlic, 2 tablespoons oil, and salt. Toss well and spread out on baking sheet.

4. Bake for 30 minutes or until cauliflower starts to brown. Remove from oven and add chopped spinach to the hot baking sheet. Toss vegetables together until spinach wilts.

5. While cauliflower is roasting, cook pasta according to directions on package. Strain and drizzle with a splash of olive oil to prevent it from sticking together.

6. Toss warm cooked pasta and roasted cauliflower mixture in a large bowl along with lemon zest, basil, nuts, and red pepper flakes. Drizzle with remaining 1 tablespoon oil and toss to coat.

7. Serve topped with extra fresh herbs or nuts. Add salt and pepper to taste.

COOK TIME: 40 MINUTES
SERVES 3–4

> Garlic contains many medicinal compounds, making it one of the most beneficial foods we can add to our diets. Adding garlic to our food increases the amount of antioxidants we consume while adding antimicrobial and immune-boosting benefits.

SHEET-PAN FISH & VEGETABLE FAJITAS

These fajitas can be served in a lettuce or cabbage wrap or as a bowl with quinoa and black or pinto beans. Add any vegetables you'd like along with avocado, hot sauce, chopped cilantro, and/or green onions. You can use any white fish, like cod, snapper, or halibut.

INGREDIENTS

1 pound white fish

1 red bell pepper, sliced into strips (optional; omit if nightshade-free)

½ red onion, sliced into half-moons

1 zucchini, sliced into matchsticks

1 teaspoon smoked paprika (optional; omit if nightshade-free)

1 teaspoon garlic powder

1 teaspoon chili powder (optional; omit if nightshade-free)

¾ teaspoon sea salt

½ teaspoon ground cumin

Lettuce or cabbage leaves for wraps

OPTIONAL TOPPINGS:

Shredded lettuce

Chopped cilantro

Shredded cabbage

Chopped green onions

Avocado

Hot sauce (omit if nightshade-free)

INSTRUCTIONS

1. Preheat oven to 350°F and line a baking sheet with parchment paper.

2. Cut fish into 2-inch strips and place in a medium-sized bowl with bell pepper, red onion, and zucchini.

3. Add smoked paprika, garlic powder, chili powder, salt, and cumin. Toss and coat well.

4. Place fish and vegetables on the baking sheet and spread out.

5. Bake for 15 minutes or until fish is cooked through and vegetables are soft.

6. Serve on a lettuce or cabbage leaf, or as a bowl topped with chopped lettuce, cilantro, and hot sauce or any other toppings you desire.

COOK TIME: 20 MINUTES
SERVES 4

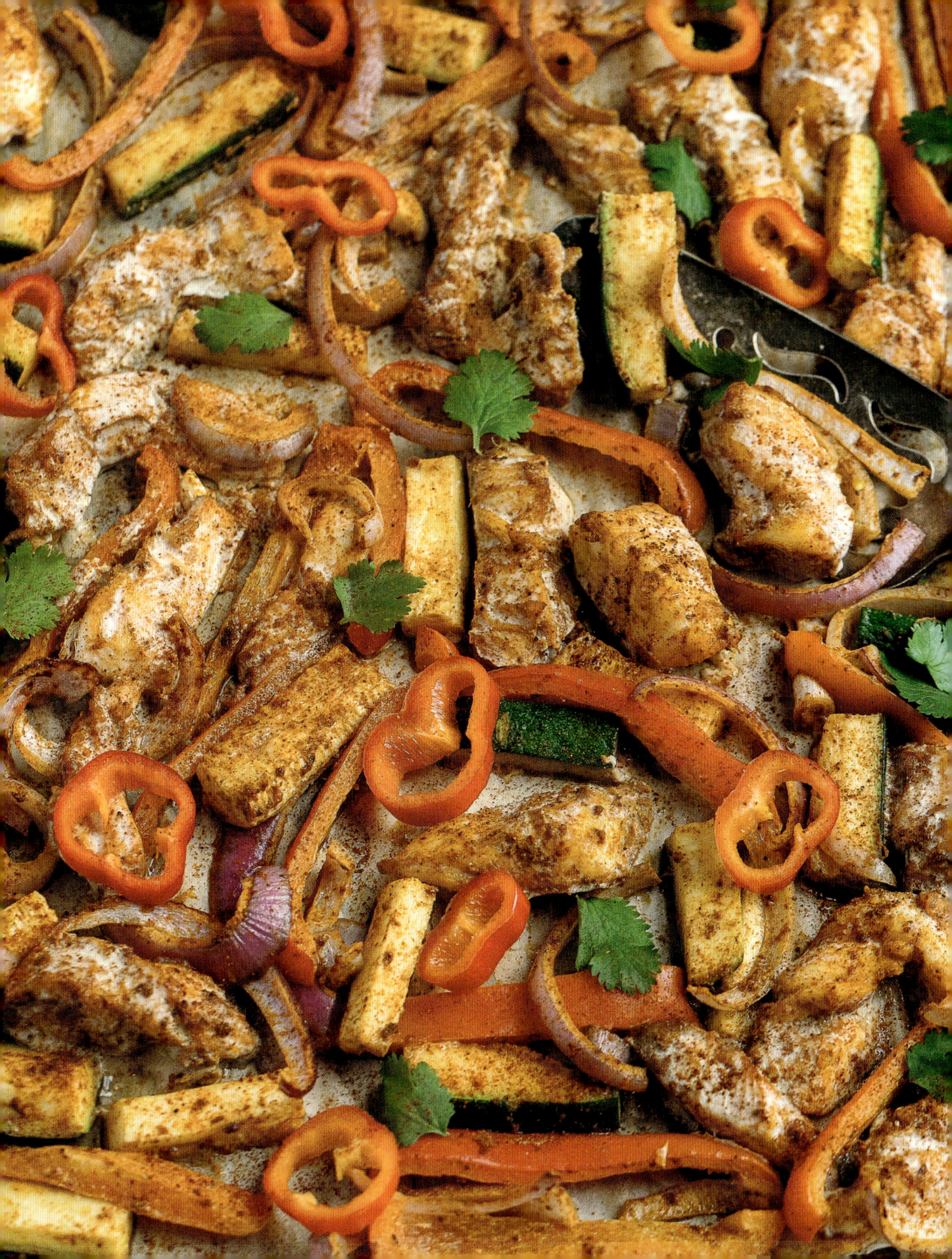

SHEPHERD'S PIE WITH CAULIFLOWER CRUST

This recipe is made with rosemary, but any herbs or spices can be used, such as thyme, parsley, or oregano. You can also use ground turkey or chicken in place of the ground lamb. Try adding extra greens or some chopped zucchini to increase the vegetable content.

INGREDIENTS

FILLING:

- 3 tablespoons avocado oil, divided
- ½ medium yellow onion, chopped
- 2 medium carrots, chopped
- 2 cups chopped button, cremini, or shiitake mushrooms
- ½ bunch chard or kale, chopped
- ½ teaspoon sea salt
- 1½ pounds grass-fed ground lamb
- ¼ cup coconut aminos
- 3–4 tablespoons balsamic or apple cider vinegar
- 1–2 teaspoons crushed dried rosemary, or 1 tablespoon chopped fresh rosemary
- Pinch of pepper

CRUST:

- 2 heads cauliflower, cut into 1-inch florets
- ¼ cup avocado or olive oil
- ½ teaspoon garlic powder
- ½ teaspoon sea salt

FILLING INSTRUCTIONS

1. In a medium-sized skillet, heat 2 tablespoons avocado oil on medium-high heat.

2. Add onions and a pinch of salt. Sauté until soft and translucent. Add carrots and mushrooms and sauté for an additional 3–5 minutes. Next, add chard/kale and cook until soft, about 1 minute.

3. Taste and season with salt if needed, then turn off heat and set aside.

4. In another large pan, heat remaining 1 tablespoon oil. Generously salt ground lamb, add it to preheated pan, and cook until brown, straining juices as they form.

5. Once meat is cooked through, add coconut aminos, vinegar, and rosemary. Cook for a couple of minutes, then add salt and pepper to taste.

6. Add meat to vegetable mixture and stir well to combine. Move meat and vegetable mixture to a lightly greased 9×13-inch pan and set aside while making crust.

CRUST INSTRUCTIONS

1. Preheat oven to 350°F.

2. In a large pot, add 1 inch water and bring to a boil.

3. Add cauliflower, cover and steam until soft, 7–9 minutes (be careful not to oversteam or cauliflower will be mushy).

4. Allow cauliflower to cool. Using a slotted spoon, add it to a food processor fitted with an S-blade along with oil, garlic powder, and salt. Process in batches if needed. Process cauliflower until smooth, adding small amounts of water if needed. Add to a large bowl and add extra salt, garlic powder, or oil to taste.

5. Spread cauliflower mixture over meat and vegetables to create a thin layer on top and bake at 350°F for 35–40 minutes. Turn up heat for the last 5–10 minutes to brown the top, if desired.

6. Allow shepherd's pie to cool for a few minutes. Serve warm and feel free to top with chopped fresh herbs you'd like.

COOK TIME: 1 HOUR & 30 MINUTES
SERVES 6-8

WHOLE ROASTED CHICKEN WITH VEGETABLES

This chicken is great for providing tasty leftovers for lunch during the week. Add any vegetables you'd like. Root vegetables work well, as do cauliflower and broccoli.

INGREDIENTS

1 whole chicken (3½–5 pounds)

1 small onion, chopped

2 celery stalks, chopped

5–6 garlic cloves, peeled

1 handful parsley, chopped

3–4 cups chopped vegetables, such as cauliflower, broccoli, carrots, turnips, or sweet potatoes

2–3 tablespoons olive or avocado oil, divided

1½ teaspoons sea salt, divided

2 teaspoons dried thyme

¼ cup fresh chopped herbs, such as thyme or rosemary (optional)

INSTRUCTIONS

1. Preheat oven to 425°F.

2. Place chicken in a 9×13-inch glass baking dish or roasting pan.

3. In a small bowl, mix onion, celery, and a generous pinch of salt together.

4. Place some of the mixture into the cavity of the chicken. Sprinkle the rest around chicken on bottom of pan.

5. Add garlic cloves, parsley, and chopped vegetables to a large bowl. Drizzle with 1–2 tablespoons oil and ½ teaspoon salt.

6. Add about ½ inch water to bottom of pan. Scatter vegetables around chicken.

7. Drizzle chicken with olive oil. Season generously with dried thyme and remaining 1 teaspoon salt.

8. Roast chicken for 20 minutes.

9. Turn heat down to 325°F. Roast for an additional 1 to 2 hours or until juices run clear and internal temperature is 165°F–170°F. Roasting time will depend on the size of the chicken.

> Adding thyme to your meals not only boosts the flavor of your food but also adds a medicinal quality as well. Thyme works as an antispasmodic in the gastrointestinal tract and thus helps to relieve gas, bloating, and indigestion.

COOK TIME: 1½ TO 2½ HOURS

SERVES 4–5

SOUPS & STEWS

Incorporating more soups and stews into your diet is a simple way to increase your intake of vitamins and minerals. Not only are soups simple to make, they are also very easy to digest. The soups and stews you find in this book are delicious, nourishing, and a great way to get more easy-to-digest fiber into your diet.

- Black Bean, Quinoa & Sweet Potato Stew
- Warming Winter Squash Soup
- Turkey Sausage Soup with Vegetables & Greens
- Golden Roasted Cauliflower Soup
- Healing Chicken "Noodle" Soup
- Anti-Inflammatory Turkey Chili
- Easy Lamb & Vegetable Stew
- Warming Turmeric, Fish & Vegetable Soup

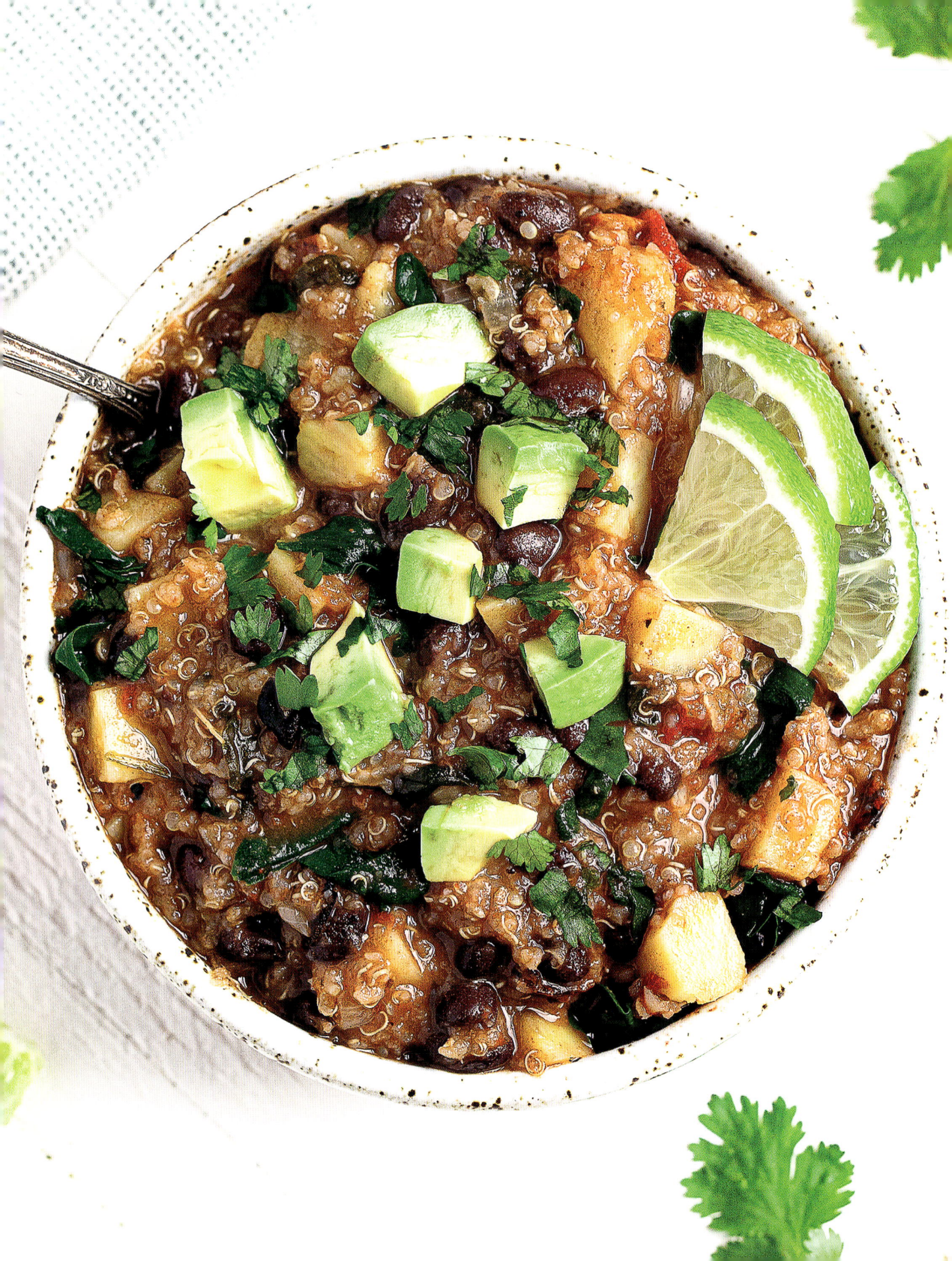

BLACK BEAN, QUINOA & SWEET POTATO STEW

This is a very easy, filling soup you can make quickly for weekday lunches. Feel free to add some extra greens if you are craving them. Rinse the quinoa well with warm water to remove the saponin, which can give it a bitter taste. Serve topped with avocado, chopped cilantro, and nightshade-free hot sauce if desired.

INGREDIENTS

- 2 tablespoons avocado or olive oil
- 1 medium yellow onion, chopped
- 3 garlic cloves, minced
- 2 medium yellow or orange sweet potatoes, peeled and cut into 1-inch cubes
- 1 cup quinoa, rinsed well with warm water and strained
- 2 (15-ounce) cans black beans, strained and rinsed
- 2 tablespoons coconut aminos
- 2 teaspoons smoked paprika (optional; omit if nightshade-free)
- 1 teaspoon ground cumin
- 1 teaspoon sea salt
- Dash of pepper (optional; omit if nightshade-free)
- 5 cups chicken or vegetable broth
- 3–4 cups chopped kale, collard greens, or spinach leaves

INSTRUCTIONS

1. In a large soup pot, heat oil on medium heat. Add onion and a pinch of salt. Stir occasionally until onion starts to caramelize, about 5–7 minutes. Add garlic and stir for 1 minute.

2. Stir in cubed sweet potatoes, rinsed quinoa, black beans, coconut aminos, smoked paprika, cumin, salt, and pepper.

3. Add broth and bring to a boil, then reduce heat to a simmer. Allow soup to simmer for 15–20 minutes or until sweet potatoes are soft and quinoa is cooked through.

4. Turn off heat and stir in chopped greens.

5. Allow soup to sit until greens are wilted. Serve topped with avocado, chopped cilantro, and hot sauce if desired.

COOK TIME: 30 MINUTES
SERVES 4–6

WARMING WINTER SQUASH SOUP

This is a delicious and warming winter soup. You can substitute any winter squash you like or use just the butternut squash. This soup is best made with chicken or vegetable broth. Add more coconut milk to taste or reserve some to drizzle on top of each serving.

INGREDIENTS

- 2 tablespoons avocado or olive oil
- 1 large onion, finely chopped
- 3 garlic cloves, minced
- 6 cups chicken or vegetable broth
- 5 cups 1-inch pieces of peeled butternut squash
- 3 cups 1-inch pieces peeled acorn squash
- 1½ teaspoons minced fresh thyme, or ¾ teaspoon dried
- 1 teaspoon ground cumin
- ½ teaspoon dried sage powder
- ½ teaspoon ground ginger
- ½ cup full-fat coconut milk
- Sea salt and black pepper

INSTRUCTIONS

1. Add oil to a large pot on medium heat.

2. Add onion, garlic, and a pinch of salt and cook until soft.

3. Add broth, both squashes, thyme, cumin, sage, and ginger. Bring to a boil, reduce heat, and simmer for 20 minutes or until squash is soft.

4. Allow soup to cool enough to puree in a blender or use an immersion blender.

5. Add soup back to pot and stir in coconut milk. Add salt and pepper to taste.

COOK TIME: 35 MINUTES
SERVES 6

> The more spices we use in our foods the better. Culinary spices like sage, ginger, thyme, and cumin have been shown to increase the nutritional value of the foods we eat. These spices can also reduce oxidative stress, support your gastrointestinal health, and boost your immune system.

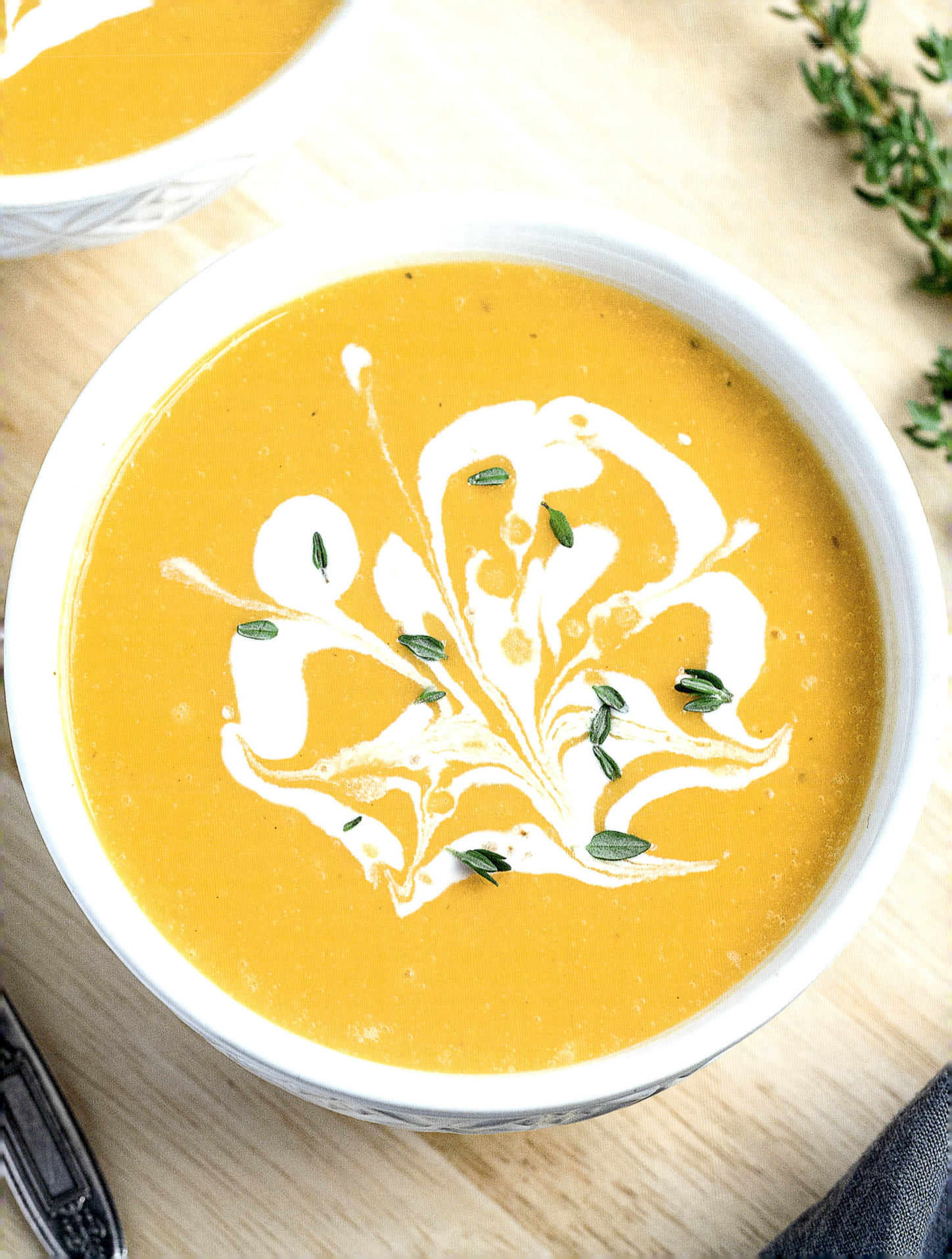

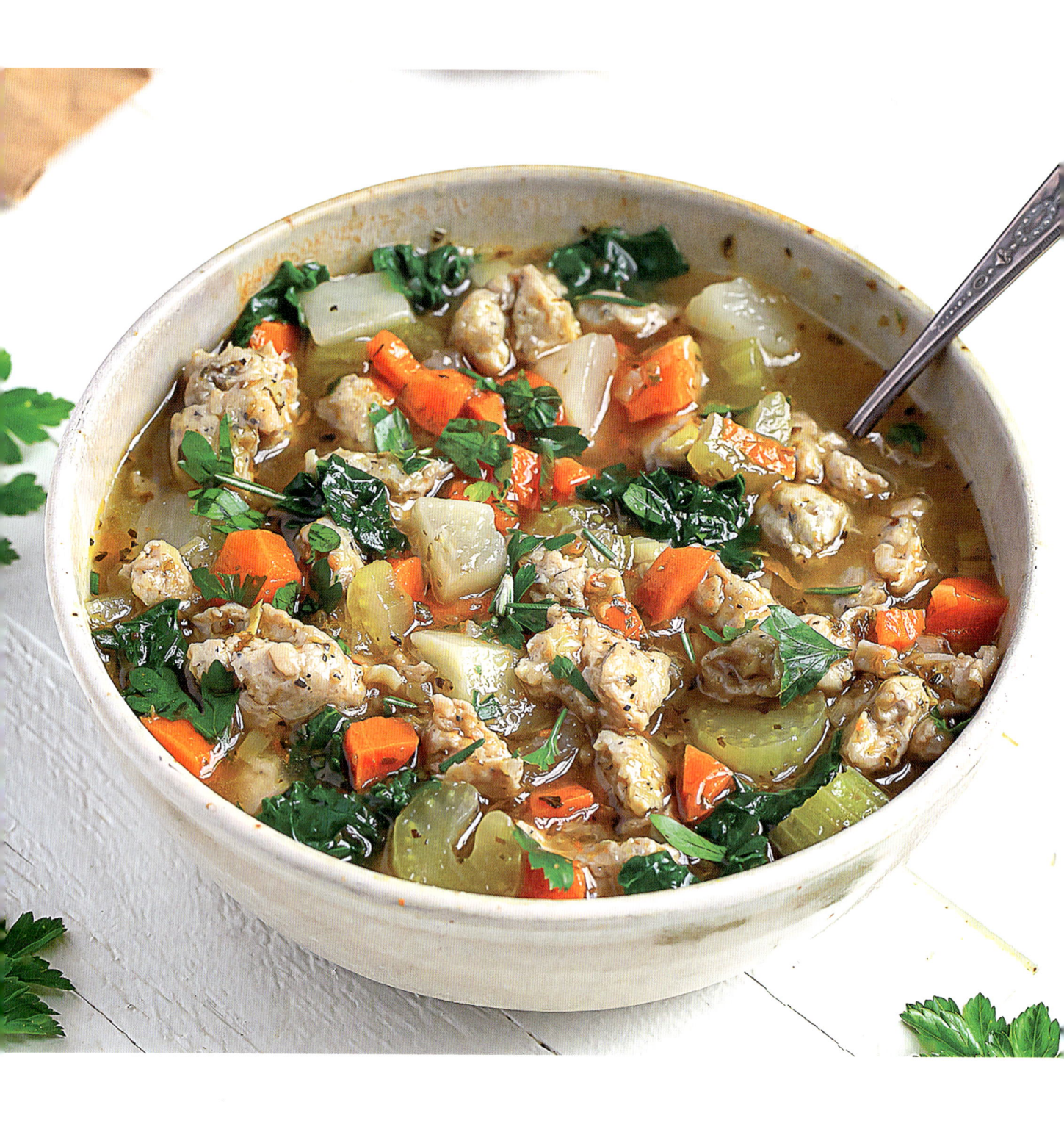

TURKEY SAUSAGE SOUP WITH VEGETABLES & GREENS

This is a delicious, warming soup to have any time of the year. Make enough for leftovers that can easily be reheated for a quick lunch. It is a full meal on its own but can also be served with a side of steamed quinoa. Store for up to 4 days in an airtight glass container in the refrigerator.

INGREDIENTS

- 2 tablespoons olive or avocado oil
- ¾ pound ground turkey sausage (homemade) or plain ground turkey (white meat, dark meat, or a combination)
- ½–¾ teaspoon sea salt, divided
- Large pinch of pepper (optional; omit if nightshade-free)
- 1 leek, chopped
- 2 garlic cloves, minced
- 1 medium turnip, peeled and cubed
- 2 celery stalks, sliced
- 2 carrots, chopped
- 1½ teaspoons Italian seasoning mix
- 4½ cups chicken broth
- 4 cups chopped kale
- Chopped parsley (optional)

INSTRUCTIONS

1. Heat oil in a large soup pot on medium heat. Crumble turkey and cook until browned and cooked through. Add ¼ teaspoon salt and a pinch of pepper. Remove cooked turkey from pot and set aside on a plate. Strain any extra liquid from pot and return to stove.

2. Add leeks and a dash of oil to pot with a pinch of salt. Cook until soft, about 5–7 minutes, then add garlic and stir in quickly.

3. Add turnips, celery, carrots, Italian seasoning, another ¼ teaspoon salt, and pepper. Cook for 3–5 minutes until vegetables start to soften, then add broth and turkey back to pot. Bring to a boil and simmer for 15 minutes until all vegetables are soft.

4. Add chopped kale. Cook until kale is bright green and soft.

5. Add salt and pepper to taste. Serve topped with chopped parsley, if desired.

COOK TIME: 30 MINUTES
SERVES 4

GOLDEN ROASTED CAULIFLOWER SOUP

This easy soup is a great way to incorporate more vegetables into your diet. Roasting the cauliflower brings out the sweetness, and the added turmeric is great for its anti-inflammatory properties and beautiful color. Add extra lime or salt to taste and top with chopped fresh mint, cilantro, or parsley.

INGREDIENTS

- 1 medium cauliflower, cut into 1-inch pieces
- 5 tablespoons avocado oil, divided
- ¾ teaspoon sea salt, divided
- ½ teaspoon turmeric powder
- 1 medium onion, chopped
- 2 garlic cloves, minced
- 2 carrots, chopped
- 1 celery stalk, chopped
- 4 cups chicken or vegetable broth
- 1 (13.5-ounce) can coconut milk
- 2–3 teaspoons fresh ginger
- 1 tablespoon lime juice
- 1 tablespoon finely chopped fresh parsley, mint, or cilantro

INSTRUCTIONS

1. Preheat oven to 425°F and line a baking sheet with parchment paper.

2. Place cauliflower on baking sheet and drizzle 3 tablespoons avocado oil over it. Sprinkle ½ teaspoon salt and turmeric and toss until cauliflower is evenly coated. Spread evenly on baking sheet.

3. Bake for 20–25 minutes until cauliflower is golden brown. Remove from oven and allow to sit while other soup ingredients simmer.

4. While cauliflower roasts, heat remaining 2 tablespoons oil in a large soup pot on medium heat. Add onion and a pinch of salt, cooking until translucent for 3–5 minutes.

5. Add garlic, carrots, celery, and remaining ¼ teaspoon of salt. Cook until vegetables begin to turn golden, about 10 minutes.

6. Add broth and bring to a boil, then reduce heat and simmer for 8–10 minutes until liquid starts to cook down.

7. Add coconut milk, ginger, and roasted cauliflower to pan. Simmer for an additional 2–3 minutes, then turn off heat.

8. Allow soup ingredients to cool. Transfer soup to a blender with lime juice and blend until smooth. Return mixture to pot and heat until warm.

9. Adjust lime and salt to taste.

10. Serve topped with fresh cilantro, mint, or parsley if desired.

COOK TIME: 45–50 MINUTES
SERVES 6

Cauliflower is a vegetable found in the brassica family that has many antioxidant and anti-inflammatory properties which aid the body in lowering oxidative stress. It's also a good source of fiber which helps reduce constipation, which is one of the leading causes of inflammation in the body.

HEALING CHICKEN "NOODLE" SOUP

This is a great soup to have on hand during the winter months or when you want to build up your immune system. You can add extra vegetables such as turnips or parsnips or some chopped green kale. Serve this soup with a side salad for a full meal or as is garnished with fresh herbs like parsley, rosemary, or fresh thyme.

INGREDIENTS

- 2 bone-in chicken breasts
- 2 bone-in chicken legs/thighs
- 1 large onion, chopped
- 4 medium carrots, sliced into rounds
- 2 celery stalks, sliced
- 2 garlic cloves, minced
- 1 tablespoon grated fresh ginger
- 2–3 teaspoons sea salt
- 2 teaspoons chopped fresh rosemary, or 1 teaspoon dried
- 2 teaspoons chopped fresh thyme, or 1 teaspoon dried
- 1 teaspoon turmeric powder
- Large pinch of pepper (optional; omit if nightshade-free)
- 3 cups very thinly sliced green cabbage for the "noodles"
- Chopped fresh herbs, for garnish

INSTRUCTIONS

1. Place chicken in a large soup pot and submerge under 2 inches of water.

2. Bring water to a boil until foam forms on top. Skim foam off and discard.

3. Add onion, carrots, celery, garlic, ginger, salt, rosemary, thyme, turmeric, and pepper to pot and bring to a rolling boil, then reduce heat to a simmer. Cover pot, leaving a crack, and simmer for 1½ to 2 hours until meat begins to fall off the bone.

4. Turn off heat and remove chicken from pot. Allow chicken to cool enough to touch. Debone and place meat back in pot with cabbage.

5. Bring soup back to a rolling boil, then reduce heat to a simmer for 5–7 more minutes until cabbage softens. Turn off heat and serve warm topped with chopped fresh herbs.

COOK TIME: 2½ HOURS
SERVES 6–8

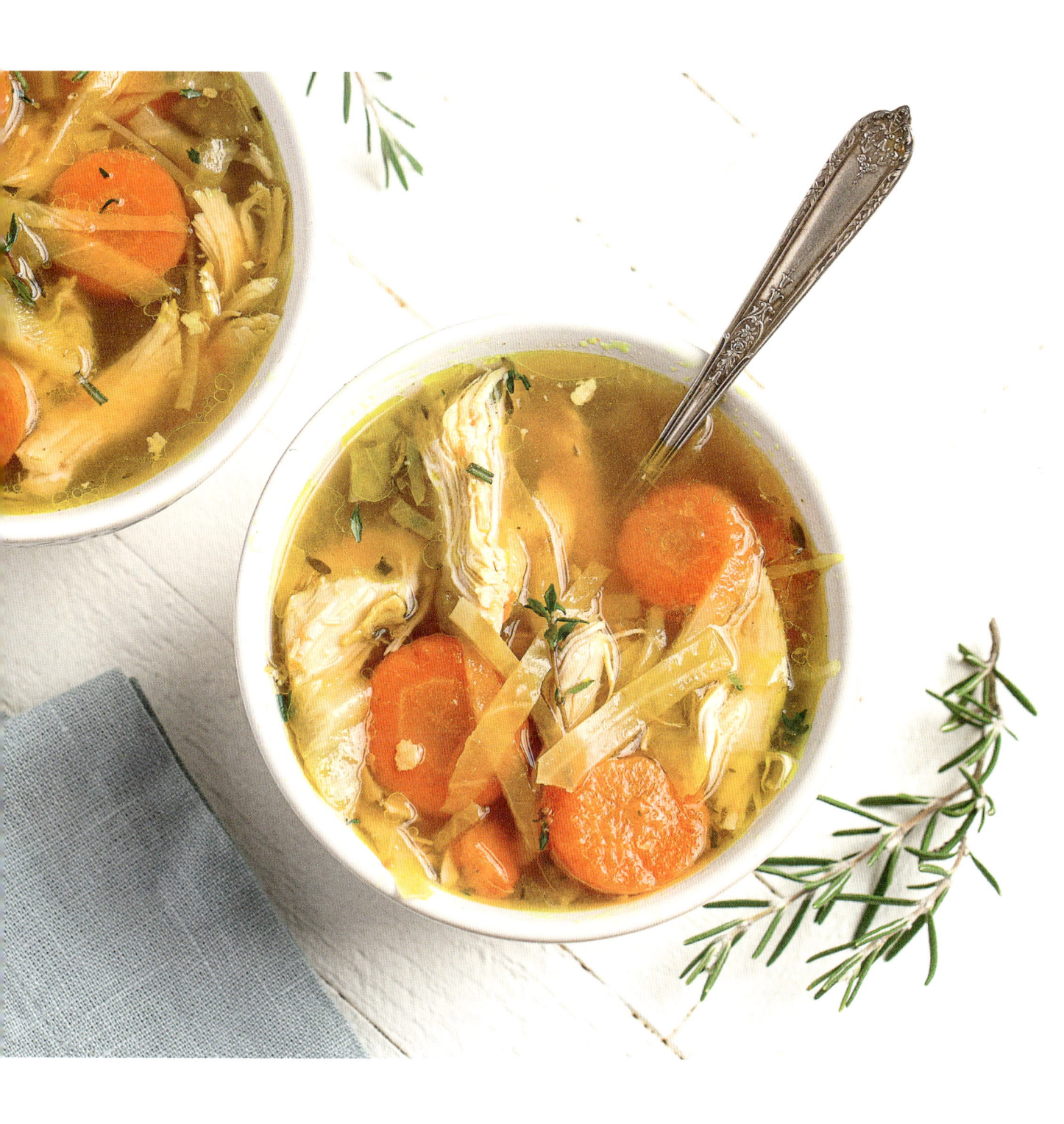

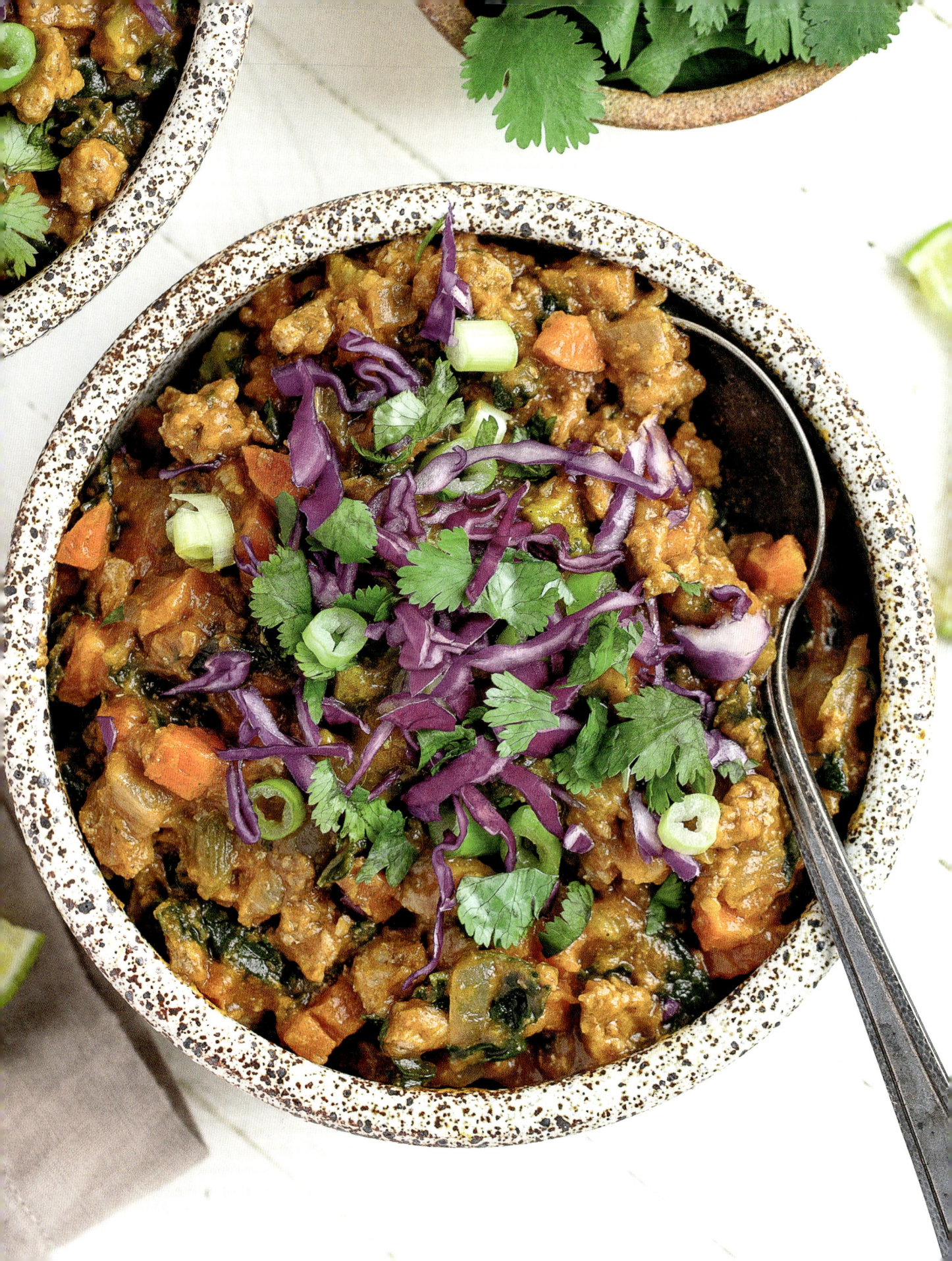

ANTI-INFLAMMATORY TURKEY CHILI

This turkey chili is ideal to have around for a quick leftover lunch or dinner. You can use white or dark meat, although dark is preferred. It is great served as is or along with the optional toppings. You can also serve the chili with Inflammatory Reset–friendly plantain chips or steamed quinoa.

INGREDIENTS

3 tablespoons avocado oil
1 small yellow onion, chopped
4 garlic cloves, minced
2 medium carrots, chopped
1 celery stalk, chopped
2 teaspoons dried oregano
1 teaspoon ground cumin
½ teaspoon cinnamon
½ teaspoon turmeric powder
½ teaspoon sea salt
½ cup coconut aminos
3 cups chicken broth

1–1½ pounds ground turkey (preferably dark meat)
1 (13.5-ounce) can organic pumpkin puree
3 cups chopped green kale

OPTIONAL TOPPINGS:
Chopped cilantro
Sliced red or green cabbage
Sliced green onions
Squeeze of lime
Sliced avocado
Diced red onion

INSTRUCTIONS

1. Heat oil in a large saucepan or soup pot on medium heat. Add onion and a pinch of salt. Cook until onion starts to soften.

2. Add garlic, carrots, celery, oregano, cumin, cinnamon, turmeric, and salt. Cook for 3–5 minutes or until vegetables start to soften.

3. Add turkey and combine well with vegetables, breaking up turkey into pieces and cooking for 8–10 minutes or until turkey is cooked through. Add coconut aminos and stir to coat for 30 seconds.

4. Add pumpkin puree and chicken broth, then bring to a boil. Reduce heat and simmer uncovered for 20 minutes.

5. Add chopped kale and simmer for an additional 2–3 minutes or until kale is soft.

6. Add additional salt or coconut aminos to taste.

7. Serve as is or top with cilantro, cabbage, green onions, lime, avocado, or red onion.

COOK TIME: 40–45 MINUTES
SERVES 4–5

EASY LAMB & VEGETABLE STEW

Super easy to make and loaded with healthy anti-inflammatory ingredients, this lamb stew is ideal served alongside a salad or steamed quinoa for a full meal. You can also add extra greens to the stew. Allow at least 2 hours for this stew to simmer. I like to start it in the afternoon so it is ready at dinnertime.

INGREDIENTS

- 1½ pounds grass-fed lamb stew meat
- 1 teaspoon sea salt
- 3 tablespoons avocado oil, divided
- 1 medium yellow onion, chopped
- 4 garlic cloves, minced
- 4 medium carrots, sliced
- 2 celery ribs, sliced
- 2 tablespoons coconut aminos
- 1 teaspoon dried thyme
- 1 teaspoon paprika (optional; omit if nightshade-free)
- ½ teaspoon cinnamon
- 4 cups chicken broth
- 3 cups chopped kale or chard

INSTRUCTIONS

1. Add lamb and sea salt to a large bowl and toss well.

2. In a 4–6 quart pot, heat 2 tablespoons avocado oil at medium-high heat until hot but not smoking.

3. Cook lamb until browned on all sides, then transfer to a bowl and set aside.

4. In the same pot on medium heat, cook onion and garlic along with remaining 1 tablespoon avocado oil for 2–3 minutes or until softened.

5. Add carrots, celery, coconut aminos, thyme, paprika, and cinnamon and cook, stirring, for 1 minute.

6. Add broth and lamb. Bring to a boil. Reduce heat and simmer, partially covered, for 2 to 2½ hours or until stew starts to thicken and lamb is very tender.

COOK TIME: 3 HOURS

SERVES 4–6

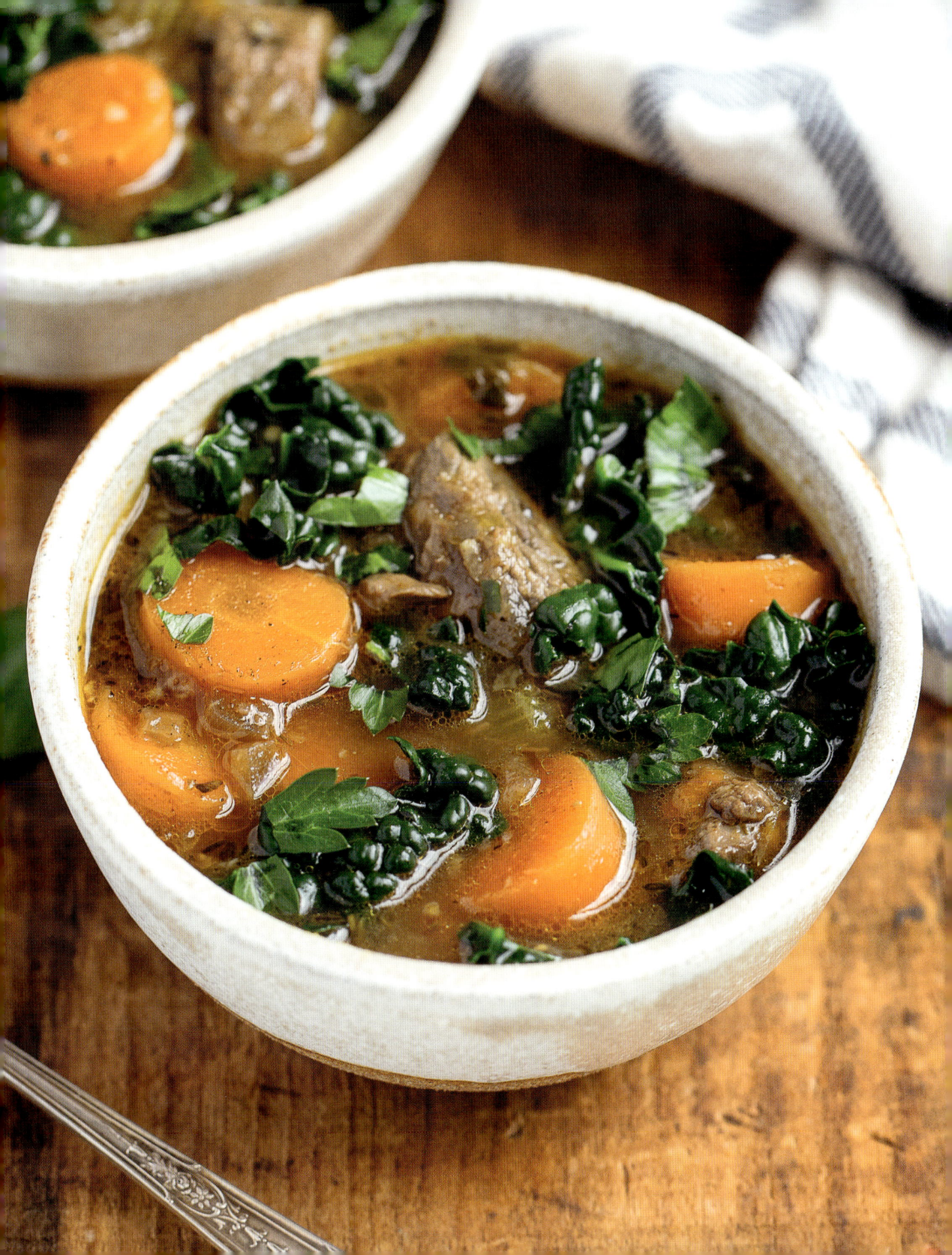

WARMING TURMERIC, FISH & VEGETABLE SOUP

This soup is easy to make and very adaptable. You can add any vegetables, substitute vegetable broth for chicken stock, add extra greens, fresh herbs, or even substitute chicken for the fish.

INGREDIENTS

2 tablespoons avocado oil
1 medium onion, chopped
2 garlic cloves, minced
2 celery stalks, sliced
1 medium parsnip, peeled and sliced
2 medium turnips, cubed
2 medium carrots, sliced
1 teaspoon dried thyme
1 teaspoon turmeric powder

½ teaspoon sea salt
4 cups chicken or vegetable stock
1 (13.5-ounce) can full-fat coconut milk
2 cups chopped kale, chard, or collard greens
1 pound wild-caught halibut or other white fish, skin removed, cut to bite-sized cubes
Black pepper
Chopped fresh herbs, such as cilantro, parsley, or dill

INSTRUCTIONS

1. Heat avocado oil in a large soup pot on medium heat. Add chopped onion and a pinch of salt. Cook until onions are soft.

2. Add celery, parsnips, turnips, carrots, thyme, turmeric, and salt. Stir to coat vegetables for 2–3 minutes and then add chicken stock and coconut milk.

3. Bring soup to a boil, then reduce heat to simmer for 15–20 minutes or until vegetables are soft.

4. Add chopped greens and halibut. Simmer for another 5–7 minutes or until fish is cooked through.

5. Add salt and pepper to taste and top with fresh herbs, if desired.

COOK TIME: 45 MINUTES
SERVES 4–6

> When it comes to lowering inflammation in the body, no spice is more beneficial than turmeric. The health benefits can be found in its curcuminoids, which are well known for boosting immunity, reducing inflammation, and keeping joint pain at bay. To maximize turmeric's benefits, add a bit of black pepper to enhance absorption. (Avoid pepper if you are nightshade-free.)

ABOUT OUR RECIPE DEVELOPER & PHOTOGRAPHER

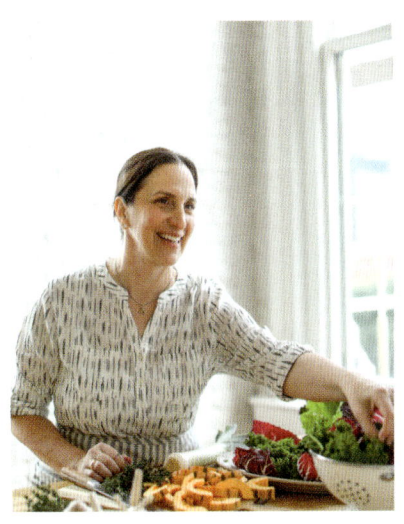

All of our recipes and photos were created by **Andrea Livingston.** Andrea is a holistic recipe developer, healthy food content creator, and food photographer based in Portland, Oregon. She creates nutrition and culinary content for a variety of functional medicine doctors, wellness practitioners, food bloggers, fitness studios, and more, collaborating behind the scenes on blogs, social media, and cookbooks.

Andrea's journey with food-as-medicine began when she needed to find health and balance in her own body and had to establish a new relationship with the foods she ate, getting to know the healing potential of each ingredient. Food truly became medicine. As she learned about the power of healing foods, she became passionate about helping other people to cultivate healthy relationships with the foods they eat and with the foods that nourish them specifically.

When she's not in the kitchen, she enjoys perusing the local farmers markets, spending time with her family, and taking long walks with her dog. You can find her at AndreaLivingston.com or @CulinaryRemedy on Instagram.

YOU CAN DO IT

The Inflammatory Reset can be a challenge, but your health is the most important aspect of your life to keep chipping away at. It may be hard to dive in entirely to the multipronged approach, and for some it's best to start with a couple of items to bring into your routine. Start small, be consistent. Implementing small changes gradually will bring some new and great things. Before you know it, 30 days will have already passed.

You can do it. With this guide, you now have the resources to enact changes within your own life that will positively impact your health.

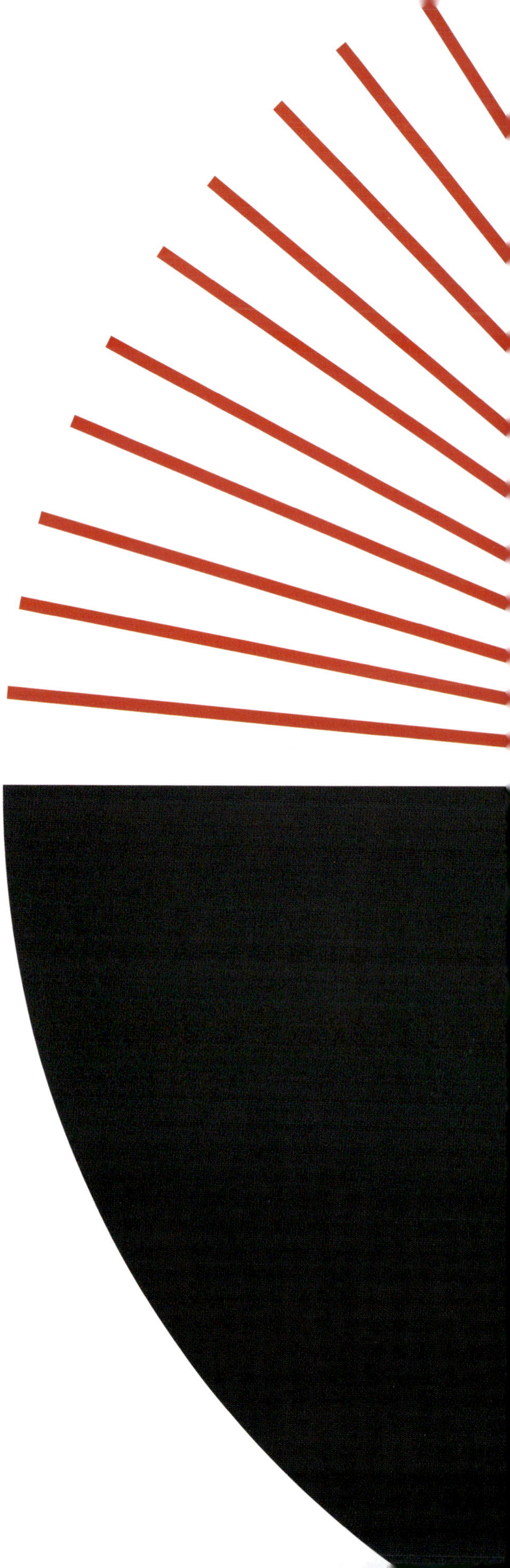

APPENDICES

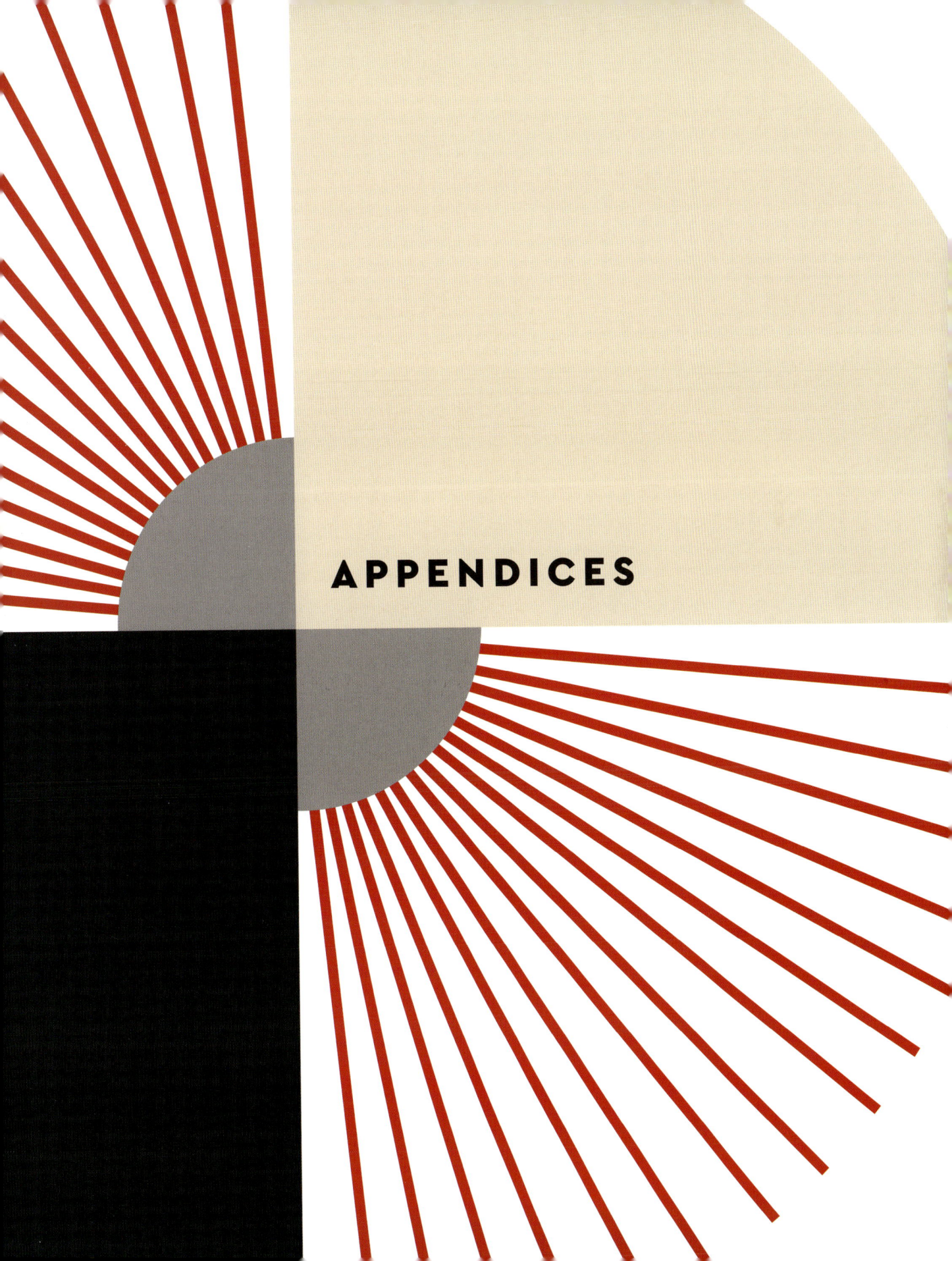

CUTTING-EDGE TESTING

Have you ever had a conventional blood test come back normal even though you suffer from fatigue, brain fog, hair loss, digestive issues, joint pain, or some other symptom? Or maybe a medical professional has prescribed something, such as an antidepressant, that hasn't worked. These are common dilemmas that many of our patients have experienced.

Standard blood tests screen for diseases instead of *trends* toward disease. But in functional medicine, blood tests assess disease risk so you can do something about a downward trend before it's too late. For instance, functional medicine practitioners can identify a risk for diabetes long before the condition occurs or explain why you have hypothyroid symptoms despite normal lab results.

The lab tests that a functional medicine practitioner recommends can be costly, but they can save you money in the long run by eliminating trial-and-error guesswork. Getting feedback from your lab tests also works wonders for compliance, helping you reach your goals faster and with more conviction.

A blood test for functional medicine is thorough. Because functional medicine practitioners look at a complete picture of physiological function, they use blood tests that include many more markers than standard tests.

For instance, many conventional doctors typically look only at blood levels of thyroid-stimulating hormone (TSH), a basic marker of thyroid function, when they suspect hypothyroidism. In functional medicine, we understand that Hashimoto's hypothyroidism is an autoimmune disease that attacks and destroys the thyroid gland. Therefore, we also order blood tests that measure thyroid antibodies, a marker of autoimmunity, to identify imbalances such as under-conversion problems, protein binding problems, and other markers that pinpoint the exact mechanism driving thyroid symptoms and problems.

APPENDICES

You can test for inflammation by asking your doctor to run the following blood markers. If these markers come back high, you can implement the Inflammatory Reset and retest every 30 days to see if you're making a difference with your overall inflammation. Use the laboratory reference ranges to evaluate most of these:

1. C-reactive protein (CRP): 0–3, hs-CRP (high-sensitivity CRP).

2. Homocysteine: <7.

3. Ferritin:
    a. Anything above 122 in premenopausal women and above 263 in post-menopausal women is an indication of inflammation.
    b. Anything above 236 in men is an indication of inflammation.

4. Lactate dehydrogenase (LDH): 140–180. (If outside the laboratory range, run an LD isoenzymes test to see which tissue is affected.)

5. Uric acid (linked to acute phase reactants and induces hepatic inflammatory molecules):
    a. Women: 3.2–5.5
    b. Men: 3.7–6.0

6. Sed rate, or erythrocyte sedimentation rate (ESR): Use lab range. (Detects alteration of blood proteins, which typically indicates inflammation.)

7. High-density lipoprotein (HDL): Functional range: 55–100. Levels over 85 may suggest inflammation (acute phase reactant).

INFLAMMATORY-FOCUSED CLINICS

RedRiver Health and Wellness is a series of clinics I founded to help people discover the sources of their inflammation and manage it. We provide the cutting-edge testing mentioned in the previous section so that people can learn more about their inflammation. Additionally, our chiropractic physicians can help you start the Inflammatory Reset and address any other needs or questions you might have so you can get on track to reducing your inflammation and feeling great.

IDAHO

Boise
RedRiver Health and Wellness Center
3405 E. Overland Road
Suite 110
Meridian, ID 83642
(208) 314-1734

NEVADA

Henderson
RedRiver Health and Wellness Center
8935 South Pecos Road
Suite 21B
Henderson, NV 89074
(702) 323-5507

APPENDICES

NEW MEXICO

Albuquerque
RedRiver Health and Wellness Center
7930 Wyoming Blvd NE, Suite B
Albuquerque, NM 87109
(505) 207-3591

UTAH

Logan
RedRiver Health and Wellness Center
1454 N 200 E, Suite 250 A
Logan, UT 84341
(435) 265-4287

South Jordan
RedRiver Health and Wellness Center
10965 S River Front Pkwy
South Jordan, UT 84095
(801) 797-3682

Springville
RedRiver Health and Wellness Center
1851 W 500 S, Suite C2
Springville, UT 84663
(801) 609-7935

St. George
RedRiver Health and Wellness Center
1490 Foremaster Dr, #130
St. George, UT 84790
(435) 236-2886

RECOMMENDED PRODUCTS & TOOLS

In building this book for over a decade, I've practiced and exercised a lot of the methods with various tools and other equipment in order to get the best results in reducing inflammation. Read on for some recommendations that have produced the best outcomes for my patients and even myself.

To see some of my favorite products online with links, use the following QR code.

AIR & WATER

Clearly Filtered Water Filters
With pitchers, under-sink filters, and even water bottles, you can filter out BPA & BPS from your tap for drinking water and for cooking. We have a few of these convenient and high-quality water filters in our homes for daily use.

AquaTru Water Purifier
AquaTru countertop purifiers take your tap water and purify it without any installations. It lasts long and the water tastes great, but I like it because it removes more than 80 contaminants from our water, including, lead, arsenic, PFAS, fluoride, chlorine, and nitrates.

APPENDICES

AirDoctor Air Purifiers
I have a few of these in my house because they are the most effective air filter and do so quietly.

KITCHEN & COOKWARE

Pyrex Glass Storage
Use Pyrex glass storage containers instead of plastic containers like Tupperware to reduce your exposure to BPA & BPS.

Cast-Iron, 100% Ceramic & High-Quality Cookware
Avoid Teflon and generic nonstick. These three alternatives to cookware provide various ways to cook food to avoid phthalates.

Redmond Real Salt
You might think salt is salt, but Redmond Real Salt doesn't have any artificial additives or pollutants. Straight from nature—specifically from a seabed in Utah—this salt is pure, unprocessed, and full of nutritional benefits.

Redmond Re-Lyte Hydration
With essential electrolytes—tiny particles that carry electric currents and hydrate your cells—Re-Lyte ensures your whole body is hydrated and keeps your muscles working at their best levels.

Force of Nature
Clean your house the clean way. Force of Nature makes toxin-free multipurpose cleaners, not to mention reusable cloths, so you can avoid toxins and be environmentally friendly.

Unbleached Paper Products
There are a variety of unbleached paper products (paper towels, parchment paper, tampons, sanitary pads, coffee filters, etc.) that you can and should use to avoid dioxins.

THE INFLAMMATORY RESET

GARDENING

Avenger Organic Weed Killer
Instead of buying the glyphosate-full Roundup, use this organic, glyphosate-free weed killer in your backyard.

Sunday Garden Products
Modern lawn care uses millions upon millions of pounds of pesticides annually. Sunday garden products use "antiquated" methods: guidance and custom nutrients to cultivate healthy soil and support the ecosystem in a sustainable way.

SKIN CARE, COSMETICS & BODY APPLICATORS

Just Ingredients
From Karalynne Call's famous podcast and Instagram page, she curates a catalog of all-natural beauty and self-care products, including lip balms, face scrubs and serums, deodorant, and dry shampoos. You can find them at the following QR code.

DIME Beauty
Clean, effective, and affordable, these beauty products from DIME Beauty are wonderful and luxurious. Additionally, they have wellness and skin care products that are very effective.

Beauty by Earth

Beauty by Earth makes a lot of cosmetic and care products that are great to avoid phthalates. Some of them include moisturizers, makeup removers, deodorants, facial oils, lip balms, sunscreen, and more.

Sustain Natural and Coconu Lubricants

These nontoxic lubricants are all natural and good for intercourse and menstruation to avoid parabens.

Cora Organic Tampons

What you put in your body matters. Cora makes comfortable tampons from organic cotton, without all the pesticides, dioxins, fragrances, or chlorine that many other companies use.

EQUIPMENT FOR ANTI-INFLAMMATORY EXERCISES

Tongue Depressors

A variety of cheap options can be found online to help you stimulate the vagus nerve and reduce inflammation.

Cold Plunge Tubs

If you're serious about cold-water therapy, I use a cold plunge tub in my home and at my office. There are a variety of great cold-water immersion options on the market, but I recommend this one because it is one of the more affordable ones. It also cleans the water with UV light and moves the water while you're submerged, which creates a much colder immersion environment.

Alpha-Stim Training

I recommend any of the Alpha-Stim products from their site at alpha-stim.com. They may seem a little costly, but if your inflammation is severe, Alpha-Stim can be a nice extra step to add to your daily repertoire of exercises to reduce inflammation.

THE INFLAMMATORY RESET

DIETARY SUPPLEMENTS, FOOD & NUTRITION

Just Ingredients

In addition to self-care products, Karalynne Call offers foods, pre- and post-workout items, and supplements made from real ingredients for better health, some of which we've collaborated on. Check them out at the following QR code.

PalmaVita Therapeutics

We've used these formulas at RedRiver for the last fourteen years, and our patients have had tremendous benefits from them. Try the QR code or visit my site at PalmaVita.com.

ENDNOTES

INTRODUCTION

Page

1   *it is single-handedly contributing to more chronic health conditions than any other factor and impacting countless lives:* David Furman et al., "Chronic Inflammation in the Etiology of Disease across the Life Span," *Nature Medicine* 25, no. 12 (December 2019): 1822–32, https://doi.org/10.1038/s41591-019-0675-0.

1   *We all live inflammatory lifestyles:* Mark Guinter et al., "Abstract 596: Association between an Empirically-Derived Inflammatory Lifestyle Score and Incident Colorectal Cancer," *Cancer Research* 79, no. 13 Supplement (2019): 596, https://doi.org/10.1158/1538-7445.AM2019-596; Alison N. Thorburn, Laurence Macia, and Charles R. Mackay, "Diet, Metabolites, and 'Western-Lifestyle' Inflammatory Diseases," *Immunity* 40, no. 6 (June 2014): 833–42, https://doi.org/10.1016/j.immuni.2014.05.014.

1   *We are overly stressed:* Andrea H. Weinberger et al., "Trends in Depression Prevalence in the USA from 2005 to 2015: Widening Disparities in Vulnerable Groups," *Psychological Medicine* 48, no. 8 (2018): 1308–15, https://doi.org/10.1017/S0033291717002781.

1   *our food is overly processed and full of sugar:* Ian A. Myles, "Fast Food Fever: Reviewing the Impacts of the Western Diet on Immunity," *Nutrition Journal* 13, no. 1 (2014): 1–17, https://doi.org/10.1186/1475-2891-13-61.

ENDNOTES

1 *Inflammation underlies most chronic diseases today, from diabetes:* Furman et al., "Chronic Inflammation in the Etiology of Disease," 1822–32.

1 *to thyroid issues:* Yoichi Ichikawa et al., "Altered Equilibrium between Cortisol and Cortisone in Plasma in Thyroid Dysfunction and Inflammatory Diseases," *Metabolism* 26, no. 9 (1977): 989–97, https://doi.org/10.1016/0026-0495(77)90016-6.

1 *to Alzheimer's:* Tony Wyss-Coray and Joseph Rogers, "Inflammation in Alzheimer Disease—a Brief Review of the Basic Science and Clinical Literature," *Cold Spring Harbor Perspectives in Medicine* 2, no. 1 (2012): a006346, https://doi.org/10.1101/cshperspect.a006346.

1 *causes issues such as fatigue:* Karine Louati and Francis Berenbaum, "Fatigue in Chronic Inflammation—a Link to Pain Pathways," *Arthritis Research & Therapy* 17, 254E, https://doi.org/10.1186/s13075-015-0784-1.

1 *depression:* Patricia A. Zunszain, Nilay Hepgul, and Carmine M. Pariante, "Inflammation and Depression," *Current Topics in Behavioral Neurosciences* 14 (2013): 135–51, https://doi.org/10.1007/7854_2012_211.

1 *hormonal difficulties:* Roma Pahwa et al., *Chronic Inflammation*, (Treasure Island, FL: StatPearls Publishing, 2023), https://www.ncbi.nlm.nih.gov/books/NBK493173/.

1 *chronic pain:* Ashish S. Kaushik, Larissa J. Strath, and Robert E. Sorge, "Dietary Interventions for Treatment of Chronic Pain: Oxidative Stress and Inflammation," *Pain and Therapy* 9, no. 2 (2020): 487–98, https://doi.org/10.1007/s40122-020-00200-5.

1 *gut problems:* Luxian Zeng et al., "Trends in Processed Meat, Unprocessed Red Meat, Poultry, and Fish Consumption in the United States, 1999–2016," *Journal of the Academy of Nutrition and Dietetics* 119, no. 7 (July 2019): 1085–1098.e12, https://doi.org/10.1016/j.jand.2019.04.004.

THE INFLAMMATORY RESET

WHAT IS INFLAMMATION?

6 *Inflammation is directly tied to the immune system and acts as a built-in protective physiological response:* Geert W. Schmid-Schönbein, "Analysis of Inflammation," *Annual Review of Biomedical Engineering* 8, no. 1 (1 August 2006): 93–131, https://doi.org/10.1146/annurev.bioeng.8.061505.095708.

6 *Our cells are hardwired with pattern recognition receptors:* Osamu Takeuchi and Shizuo Akira, "Pattern Recognition Receptors and Inflammation," *Cell* 140, no. 6 (2010): 805–20, https://doi.org/10.1016/j.cell.2010.01.022.

6 *But when these inflammatory pathways are triggered frequently—and without outside danger—they can aggravate and destroy the tissue around them, creating even more inflammation:* M. Fukata and M. Arditi, "The Role of Pattern Recognition Receptors in Intestinal Inflammation," *Mucosal Immunology* 6, no. 3 (May 2013): 451–63, https://doi.org/10.1038/mi.2013.13; Si Ming Man, Nadeem O. Kaakoush, and Hazel M. Mitchell, "The Role of Bacteria and Pattern-Recognition Receptors in Crohn's Disease," *Nature Reviews. Gastroenterology & Hepatology* 8, no. 3 (2011): 152–68, https://doi.org/10.1038/nrgastro.2011.3; Michelle A. Sugimoto et al., "Resolution of Inflammation: What Controls Its Onset?," *Frontiers in Immunology* 7, 160 (April 2016), https://doi.org/10.3389/fimmu.2016.00160.

HOW CAN INFLAMMATION AFFECT YOU?

7 *There are a multitude of conditions and symptoms you or a loved one can face from inflammation, and each of these areas can lead to further problems down the line, such as cancer*
Mark Guinter et al., "Abstract 596: Association between an Empirically-Derived Inflammatory Lifestyle Score and Incident Colorectal Cancer," *Cancer Research* 79, no. 13 Supplement (2019): 596, https://doi.org/10.1158/1538-7445.AM2019-596; Alison N. Thorburn, Laurence Macia, and Charles R. Mackay, "Diet, Metabolites, and 'Western-Lifestyle' Inflammatory Diseases," *Immunity* 40, no. 6 (June 2014): 833–42, https://doi.org/10.1016/j.immuni.2014.05.014.

ENDNOTES

7 *autism*
Dario Siniscalco et al., "Inflammation and Neuro-Immune Dysregulations in Autism Spectrum Disorders," *Pharmaceuticals (Basel, Switzerland)* 11, no. 2 (2018): 56, https://doi.org/10.3390/ph11020056.

7 *infertility*
Ashok Agarwal et al., "Role of Oxidative Stress, Infection and Inflammation in Male Infertility," *Andrologia* 50, no. 11 (2018): e13126, https://doi.org/ 10.1111/and.13126; Gülden Halis and Aydin Arici, "Endometriosis and Inflammation in Infertility," *Annals of the New York Academy of Sciences* 1034 (2004): 300–15, https://doi.org/10.1196/annals.1335.032.

7 *Studies show chronic inflammation and the factors that contribute to it—particularly high blood sugar and insulin resistance—underlie the most common health disorders and diseases today.*
David Furman et al., "Chronic Inflammation in the Etiology of Disease across the Life Span," *Nature Medicine* 25, no. 12 (December 2019): 1822–32, https://doi.org/10.1038/s41591-019-0675-0.

7 *The kinds of inflammation your body can experience may seem overwhelming, but I want to show how commonplace inflammation is*
Dawn E. Alley et al., "Socioeconomic Status and C-Reactive Protein Levels in the US Population: NHANES IV," *Brain, Behavior, and Immunity* 20, no. 5 (September 2006): 498–504, https://doi.org/10.1016/j.bbi.2005.10.003.

HOW CAN INFLAMMATION AFFECT YOU?: BRAIN, COGNITION & INFLAMMATION

7 *more chronic inflammation reduces all neurotransmitter conduction.*
Andrew H Miller et al., "Cytokine Targets in the Brain: Impact on Neurotransmitters and Neurocircuits," *Depression and Anxiety* 30, no. 4 (2013): 297–306, https://doi.org/10.1002/da.22084.

7 *One of the most common symptoms [of inflammation] is brain fog.*
Michelle L. Byrne, Sarah Whittle, and Nicholas B. Allen, "The Role of Brain Structure and Function in the Association Between Inflammation and Depressive Symptoms: A Systematic Review," *Psychosomatic Medicine* 78, no. 4 (May 2016): 389–400, https://doi.org/10.1097/PSY.0000000000000311.

7   *Other brain-based symptoms of inflammation can include depression, low motivation, memory loss, clumsiness, and irritability.*
    Byrne, "The Role of Brain Structure and Function," 389–400.

7   *What's worse, these symptoms indicate your brain may be aging too fast, putting you at a higher risk for brain-degenerative diseases such as dementia and Alzheimer's.*
    Victoria E. Johnson et al., "Inflammation and White Matter Degeneration Persist for Years after a Single Traumatic Brain Injury," *Brain* 136, pt 1 (2013): 28–42, https://doi.org/10.1093/brain/aws322.

HOW CAN INFLAMMATION AFFECT YOU?: GUT HEALTH

8   *Chronic inflammation promotes intestinal permeability, also known as leaky gut*
    Alessio Fasano, "All Disease Begins in the (Leaky) Gut: Role of Zonulin-Mediated Gut Permeability in the Pathogenesis of Some Chronic Inflammatory Diseases," *F1000Research* 9, F1000 Faculty Rev-69 (2020), https://doi.org/10.12688/f1000research.20510.1.; Lisa Rizzetto et al., "Connecting the Immune System, Systemic Chronic Inflammation and the Gut Microbiome: The Role of Sex," *Journal of Autoimmunity* 92 (2018): 12–34, https://doi.org/10.1016/j.jaut.2018.05.008.

8   *[Leaky gut] increases the likelihood of gut infections, gut inflammation*
    Alessio Fasano, "All Disease Begins in the (Leaky) Gut," F1000 Faculty Rev-69; Rizzetto et al., "Connecting the Immune System," 12–34.

8   *[Leaky gut in turn increases the likelihood of] food intolerances*
    Aziz Koleilat, "Food Intolerance," *Biomedical Journal of Scientific & Technical Research* 1, no. 2 (July 2017), https://doi.org/10.26717/BJSTR.2017.01.000190.

8   *sufficient stomach acid actually **prevents** acid reflux in most cases and is vital to healthy gut and immune function.*
    S. J. Spechler, "Are We Underestimating Acid Reflux?," *Gut* 53, no. 2 (February 2004): 162–63, https://doi.org/10.1136/gut.2003.025205; Jonathan V. Wright and Lane Lenard, *Why Stomach Acid Is Good for You: Natural Relief from Heartburn, Indigestion, Reflux and GERD* (Lanham, Maryland: Rowman & Littlefield, 2001).

ENDNOTES

8 *Inflammation may inhibit the production of stomach acid*
K. E. McColl, E el-Omar, and D. Gillen, "Interactions between H. Pylori Infection, Gastric Acid Secretion and Anti-Secretory Therapy," *British Medical Bulletin* 54, no. 1 (1998): 121–38, https://doi.org/10.1093/oxfordjournals.bmb.a011663.

8 *can cause numerous gut disorders as well as poor protein absorption.*
Yan Y. Lam et al., "Role of the Gut in Visceral Fat Inflammation and Metabolic Disorders," *Obesity*, 19 (2011): 2113–2120, https://doi.org/10.1038/oby.2011.68.

HOW CAN INFLAMMATION AFFECT YOU?: HORMONE IMBALANCES

9 *In women, high inflammation is associated with symptoms that range from hair loss*
Enrico Carmina et al., "Female Pattern Hair Loss and Androgen Excess: A Report from the Multidisciplinary Androgen Excess and PCOS Committee," *The Journal of Clinical Endocrinology and Metabolism* 104, no. 7 (2019): 2875–91, https://doi.org/10.1210/jc.2018-02548.

9 *[high inflammation is associated with] infertility*
Kathiuska J. Kriedt, Ali Alchami, and Melanie C. Davies, "PCOS: Diagnosis and Management of Related Infertility," *Obstetrics, Gynaecology & Reproductive Medicine* 29, no. 1 (2019): 1–5, https://doi.org/10.1016/j.ogrm.2018.12.001.

9 *[high inflammation is associated with] complications in childbirth*
Krzysztof Katulski et al., "Pregnancy Complications in Polycystic Ovary Syndrome Patients," *Gynecological Endocrinology* 31, no. 2 (2015): 87–91, https://doi.org/10.3109/09513590.2014.974535.

9 *[high inflammation is associated with] an increased risk of autism*
Adriana Cherskov et al., "Polycystic Ovary Syndrome and Autism: A Test of the Prenatal Sex Steroid Theory," *Translational Psychiatry* 8, no. 1 (2018): 136, https://doi.org/10.1038/s41398-018-0186-7.

9   *[high inflammation is associated with] allergies, and other health challenges in their offspring.*
    Sabahat Rasool and Duru Shah, "Polycystic Ovary Syndrome (PCOS) Transition at Menopause," *Journal of Mid-Life Health* 12, no. 1 (2021): 30–32, https://doi.org/10.4103/jmh.jmh_37_21.

9   *Women who experience symptoms of dysregulated hormones as a result of high systemic inflammation also are at risk of experiencing a more difficult transition from perimenopause to menopause.*
    Rasool, "Polycystic Ovary Syndrome (PCOS) Transition at Menopause," 30–32.

HOW CAN INFLAMMATION AFFECT YOU?: LIVER & GALLBLADDER

9   *Your liver and gallbladder are vital organs for healthy digestion and detoxification.*
    D. M. Grant, "Detoxification Pathways in the Liver," *Journal of Inherited Metabolic Disease*, 14, no. 4 (1991): 421–30, https://doi.org/10.1007/BF01797915; Arlin B. Rogers and Renee Z. Dintzis, "Liver and Gallbladder," in *Comparative Anatomy and Histology* (London: Elsevier, 2012), 193–201, https://doi.org/10.1016/B978-0-12-381361-9.00013-5.

9   *Inflammation causes both to become sluggish and contributes to gallstones in the gallbladder.*
    Grant, "Detoxification Pathways in the Liver," 421–30; Rogers and Dintzis, "Liver and Gallbladder," 193–201.

9   *When these organs aren't at proper functional levels, their ability to clear toxins and metabolized hormones in the body is hampered, increasing the overall toxicity in your body*
    Karina Jordan et al., "Gastrointestinal Toxicity, Systemic Inflammation, and Liver Biochemistry in Allogeneic Hematopoietic Stem Cell Transplantation," *Biology of Blood and Marrow Transplantation* 23, no. 7 (2017): 1170–76, https://doi.org/10.1016/j.bbmt.2017.03.021.

ENDNOTES

9   *the overall toxicity in your body, which can lead to its own set of problems, including hormonal imbalances, infertility, and weight loss resistance.*
Sheba Jarvis, Catherine Williamson, and Charlotte L. Bevan. "Liver X Receptors and Male (In)fertility." *International Journal of Molecular Sciences* 20.21 (2019): 5379. https://doi.org/10.3390/ijms20215379

HOW CAN INFLAMMATION AFFECT YOU?: WEIGHT GAIN & INFLAMMATION

10 *Weight gain and weight loss resistance are often problematic issues for people with chronic inflammation.*
Andrew W. Fogarty et al., "A Prospective Study of Weight Change and Systemic Inflammation over 9 y," *The American Journal of Clinical Nutrition* 87, no. 1 (2008): 30–35, https://doi.org/10.1093/ajcn/87.1.30; B. J. Nicklas et al., "Behavioural Treatments for Chronic Systemic Inflammation: Effects of Dietary Weight Loss and Exercise Training," *Canadian Medical Association Journal* 172, no. 9 (26 April 2005): 1199–1209, https://doi.org/10.1503/cmaj.1040769.

10 *That's because inflammation slows down metabolism*
D. Aronson et al., "Obesity Is the Major Determinant of Elevated C-Reactive Protein in Subjects with the Metabolic Syndrome," *International Journal of Obesity and Related Metabolic Disorders* 28, no. 5 (2004): 674–79, https://doi.org/10.1038/sj.ijo.0802609.

10 *shuts down cellular receptor sites for fat-burning hormones*
T. Guzik, D. Mangalat, and R. Korbut, "Adipocytokines: Novel Link between Inflammation and Vascular Function?" *Journal of Physiology and Pharmacology* 57, no. 4 (2006): 505–28, https://pubmed.ncbi.nlm.nih.gov/17229978/.

10 *stalls muscle building.*
Wenjun Yang and Ping Hu, "Skeletal Muscle Regeneration Is Modulated by Inflammation," *Journal of Orthopaedic Translation* 13 (February 2018): 25–32, https://doi.org/10.1016/j.jot.2018.01.002.

HOW CAN INFLAMMATION AFFECT YOU?: BLOOD SUGAR CRASHES

10 *Inflammation causes slow uptake, poor utilization, and inefficient elimination of glucose by the cells, all of which makes people more prone to blood sugar crashes.*
Steven E. Shoelson, Jongsoon Lee, and Allison B. Goldfine, "Inflammation and Insulin Resistance," *The Journal of Clinical Investigation* 116, no. 7 (2006): 1793–1801, https://doi.org/10.1172/JCI29069.

HOW CAN INFLAMMATION AFFECT YOU?: RAISING CHOLESTEROL LEVELS

10 *Because inflammation causes you to make fat more quickly than it's burned, inflammation can cause unhealthy cholesterol markers. These include high triglycerides, high cholesterol, and small, dense LDL ('bad') cholesterol.*
Alan R. Tall and Laurent Yvan-Charvet, "Cholesterol, Inflammation and Innate Immunity," *Nature Reviews Immunology* 15, no. 2 (2015): 104–16, https://doi.org/10.1038/nri3793.

10 *reversing insulin resistance often takes longer than a month.*
Blair J. O'Neill, "Effect of Low-Carbohydrate Diets on Cardiometabolic Risk, Insulin Resistance, and Metabolic Syndrome." *Current Opinion in Endocrinology, Diabetes, and Obesity* 27.5 (2020): 301–307, https://doi.org/10.1097/MED.0000000000000569.

HOW CAN INFLAMMATION AFFECT YOU?: HEART DISEASE

11 *Inflammation is now recognized as a primary cause of heart disease.*
Mohammad Madjid and James T. Willerson, "Inflammatory Markers in Coronary Heart Disease," *British Medical Bulletin* 100 (2011): 23–38, https://doi.org/10.1093/bmb/ldr043.

11 *This is because it can lead to high levels of the amino acid homocysteine, which increases the risk of heart disease, dementia, and other neurodegenerative diseases.*
Nehal M. Elsherbiny et al., "Homocysteine Induces Inflammation in

Retina and Brain," *Biomolecules* 10, no. 3 (2020): 393, https://doi.org/10.3390/biom10030393; Brian Karl Finch et al., "The Role of Discrimination and Acculturative Stress in the Physical Health of Mexican-Origin Adults," *Hispanic Journal of Behavioral Sciences* 23, no. 4 (November 2001): 399–429, https://doi.org/10.1177/0739986301234004; Mabrouka El Oudi et al., "Homocysteine and Markers of Inflammation in Acute Coronary Syndrome," *Experimental and Clinical Cardiology* 15, no. 2 (2010): e25–8.

11 *Inflammation is also associated with insulin resistance, elevated blood sugar*
Gisela Wilcox, "Insulin and Insulin Resistance," *Clinical Biochemist Reviews* 26, no. 2 (2005): 19–39, https://pubmed.ncbi.nlm.nih.gov/16278749/.

11 *dysfunction in the lining of the blood vessels*
Jian-Jun Li, and Ji-Lin Chen, "Inflammation May Be a Bridge Connecting Hypertension and Atherosclerosis." *Medical Hypotheses* 64.5 (2005): 925–929, https://doi.org/10.1016/j.mehy.2004.10.016.

11 *increased blood pressure*
Li, "Inflammation May Be a Bridge," 925–929.

11 *declining brain function.*
Sophie M. Heringa et al., "Markers of Low-Grade Inflammation and Endothelial Dysfunction Are Related to Reduced Information Processing Speed and Executive Functioning in an Older Population—the Hoorn Study," *Psychoneuroendocrinology* 40 (2014): 108–18, https://doi.org/10.1016/j.psyneuen.2013.11.011.

HOW CAN INFLAMMATION AFFECT YOU?: AUTOIMMUNE DISEASES

11 *Autoimmunity is the result of an immune system that has become overzealous, inflamed, and imbalanced.*
Anne Davidson and Betty Diamond, "Autoimmune Diseases," *New England Journal of Medicine* 345, no. 5 (2001): 340–50, https://doi.org/10.1056/NEJM200108023450506.

CAUSES OF INFLAMMATION

12 *While everyone has different triggers, the primary causes of inflammation typically fall into five major categories: dietary*
Leo Galland, "Diet and Inflammation," *Nutrition in Clinical Practice* 25, no. 6 (2010): 634–40, https://doi.org/10.1177/0884533610385703; Dario Giugliano, Antonio Ceriello, and Katherine Esposito, "The Effects of Diet on Inflammation: Emphasis on the Metabolic Syndrome," *Journal of the American College of Cardiology* 48, no. 4 (2006): 677–85, https://doi.org/10.1016/j.jacc.2006.03.052.

12 *lifestyle*
H. Kolb and T. Mandrup-Poulsen, "The Global Diabetes Epidemic as a Consequence of Lifestyle-Induced Low-Grade Inflammation," *Diabetologia* 53, no. 1 (2010): 10–20, https://doi.org/10.1007/s00125-009-1573-7.

12 *psychological*
Ruslan Medzhitov, "Origin and Physiological Roles of Inflammation," *Nature* 454, no. 7203 (2008): 428–35, https://doi.org/10.1038/nature07201.

12 *neurological*
Stephen D. Skaper et al., "An Inflammation-Centric View of Neurological Disease: Beyond the Neuron," *Frontiers in Cellular Neuroscience* 12 (2018): 72, https://doi.org/10.3389/fncel.2018.00072.

12 *and emotional.*
George P. Chrousos, "Stress, Chronic Inflammation, and Emotional and Physical Well-Being: Concurrent Effects and Chronic Sequelae," *The Journal of Allergy and Clinical Immunology* 106, no. 5 (2000): S275–91, https://doi.org/10.1067/mai.2000.110163.

CAUSES OF INFLAMMATION: DIETARY ROOTS IN INFLAMMATION

12 *Large quantities of the foods sold in our stores are ultra-processed and filled with synthetic materials.*
Hyunju Kim, Emily A. Hu, and Casey M. Rebholz, "Ultra-Processed Food

Intake and Mortality in the USA: Results from the Third National Health and Nutrition Examination Survey (NHANES III, 1988–1994)," *Public Health Nutrition* 22, no. 10 (2019): 1777–85, https://doi.org/10.1017/S1368980018003890.

12 *Autoimmunity and chronic conditions have exploded in the last 30 years*
Larissa Galastri Baraldi et al., "Consumption of Ultra-Processed Foods and Associated Sociodemographic Factors in the USA between 2007 and 2012: Evidence from a Nationally Representative Cross-Sectional Study," *BMJ Open* 8, no. 3 (2018): e020574, https://doi.org/10.1136/bmjopen-2017-020574; Kim, Hu, and Rebholz, "Ultra-Processed Food Intake and Mortality in the USA," 1777–85.

12 *The processed carbohydrates common in processed foods*
Judith Wylie-Rosett, C. J. Segal-Isaacson, and Adam Segal-Isaacson, "Carbohydrates and Increases in Obesity: Does the Type of Carbohydrate Make a Difference?" *Obesity Research* 12, Supplement 2 (2004): 124S–129S, https://doi.org/10.1038/oby.2004.277.

12 *increase blood sugar*
Viswanathan Mohan et al., "Are Excess Carbohydrates the Main Link to Diabetes & Its Complications in Asians?" *The Indian Journal of Medical Research* 148, no. 5 (2018): 531–538, https://doi.org/10.4103/ijmr.IJMR_1698_18.

12 *Processed foods are also loaded with gluten*
Jessica R. Biesiekierski, "What Is Gluten?," *Journal of Gastroenterology and Hepatology* 32, Supplement 1 (2017): 78–81, https://doi.org/10.1111/jgh.13703.

12 *[Gluten is] linked with at least 55 diseases, most of them autoimmune. While people are more aware of gluten allergies and intolerances today, most people aren't aware they have an intolerance or even have celiac disease, both of which are ubiquitous among people with chronic inflammation.*
Karin de Punder and Leo Pruimboom, "The Dietary Intake of Wheat and Other Cereal Grains and Their Role in Inflammation," *Nutrients* 5, no. 3 (2013): 771–87, https://doi.org/10.3390/nu5030771.

13 *Industrialized seed oils and hydrogenated oils—staple ingredients in processed foods—have been shown to boost inflammation*
James J. DiNicolantonio and James H. O'Keefe, "Importance of Maintaining a Low Omega-6/Omega-3 Ratio for Reducing Inflammation," *Open Heart* 5, no. 2 (2018): e000946, https://doi.org/10.1136/openhrt-2018-000946.

13 *and lead to obesity*
R. Kubant et al., "A Comparison of Effects of Lard and Hydrogenated Vegetable Shortening on the Development of High-Fat Diet-Induced Obesity in Rats," *Nutrition & Diabetes* 5, no. 12 (2015): e188, https://doi.org/10.1038/nutd.2015.40 ; Ming Lian et al., "The Anti-Obesity Effect of Instant Pu-Erh Ripe Tea in Mice with Hydrogenated Oil Diet-Induced Obesity," *Applied Mechanics and Materials*, 644 (2014): 5239–43, https://doi.org/10.4028/www.scientific.net/AMM.644-650.5239.

13 *diabetes*
Harumi Okuyama et al., "Medicines and Vegetable Oils as Hidden Causes of Cardiovascular Disease and Diabetes," *Pharmacology* 98, no. 3–4 (2016): 134–70, https://doi.org/10.1159/000446704.

13 *and brain degeneration.*
Supta Sarkar and Madhubalaji Chegu Krishnamurthi, "Nutritional, Dietary, and Lifestyle Approaches for Prevention and Management of Alzheimer's Disease," in *Role of Nutrients in Neurological Disorders* (Springer, 2022), 61–84, https://doi.org/10.1007/978-981-16-8158-5_3.

13 *These [industrial] oils are very high in omega-6 fatty acids*
James J. DiNicolantonio and James H O'Keefe, "Omega-6 Vegetable Oils as a Driver of Coronary Heart Disease: The Oxidized Linoleic Acid Hypothesis," *Open Heart* 5, no. 2 (2018): e000898, https://doi.org/10.1136/openhrt-2018-000898.

13 *Worst of all, the hydrogenated fats in many processed foods are linked with cognitive decline, heart disease, and inflammation.*
DiNicolantonio and O'Keefe, "Importance of Maintaining a Low Omega-6/Omega-3 Ratio," e000946; Sarkar and Chegu Krishnamurthi, "Nutritional, Dietary, and Lifestyle Approaches," 61–84; Walter C. Willett, "Dietary Fats and Coronary Heart Disease,"

Journal of Internal Medicine 272, no. 1 (2012): 13-24, https://doi.org/10.1111/j.1365-2796.2012.02553.x.

13 *Humans need a balance between omega-6 and omega-3 fatty acids.*
DiNicolantonio and O'Keefe, "Importance of Maintaining a Low Omega-6/Omega-3 Ratio," e000946; Sarkar and Chegu Krishnamurthi, "Nutritional, Dietary, and Lifestyle Approaches," 61-84; Willett, "Dietary Fats and Coronary Heart Disease," 13-24.

13 *Initially, it was thought that only chronic and heavy alcohol use caused damage to brain cells.*
Clive Harper, Jillian Kril, and John Daly, "Does a 'Moderate' Alcohol Intake Damage the Brain?," *Journal of Neurology, Neurosurgery & Psychiatry* 51, no. 7 (1988): 909-13, https://doi.org/10.1136/jnnp.51.7.909.

13 *New studies show that even moderate amounts of alcohol over an extended period can damage these cells.*
Marinus N. Verbaten, "Chronic Effects of Low to Moderate Alcohol Consumption on Structural and Functional Properties of the Brain: Beneficial or Not?" *Human Psychopharmacology: Clinical and Experimental* 24, no. 3 (April 2009): 199-205, https://doi.org/10.1002/hup.1022.

13 *glial cells, the protectors and brain cleaners.*
Maiken Nedergaard and Ulrich Dirnagl, "Role of Glial Cells in Cerebral Ischemia," *Glia* 50, no. 4 (June 2005): 281-86, https://doi.org/10.1002/glia.20205.

13 *The rapid destruction of neurons leads not only to impaired decision-making, mood, and behavior but also to neurodegeneration and neurodegenerative diseases such as dementia.*
Maurice Victor, "Alcoholic Dementia," *Canadian Journal of Neurological Sciences* 21, no. 2 (1994): 88-99, https://doi.org/10.1016/S0733-8619(18)30144-0.

13 *In fact, the second leading cause of dementia is alcoholic dementia. Depending on your source, alcohol accounts for 1%-10% of the dementia cases in the United States.*
Richard A Goodman et al., "Prevalence of Dementia Subtypes in United

States Medicare Fee-for-Service Beneficiaries, 2011–2013," *Alzheimer's & Dementia* 13, no. 1 (2017): 28–37, https://doi.org/10.1016/j.jalz.2016.04.00; David W. Oslin and Mark S. Cary, "Alcohol-Related Dementia: Validation of Diagnostic Criteria," *The American Journal of Geriatric Psychiatry* 11, no. 4 (2003): 441–47, https://pubmed.ncbi.nlm.nih.gov/12837673/.

CAUSES OF INFLAMMATION: INFLAMMATORY LIFESTYLES

13 *Being overly sedentary*
Joseph Henson et al., "Sedentary Time and Markers of Chronic Low-Grade Inflammation in a High Risk Population," *PloS One* 8, no. 10 (2013): e78350, https://doi.org/10.1371/journal.pone.0078350.

13 *sleeping poorly*
Sarosh J. Motivala, "Sleep and Inflammation: Psychoneuroimmunology in the Context of Cardiovascular Disease," *Annals of Behavioral Medicine* 42, no. 2 (2011): 141–52, https://doi.org/10.1007/s12160-011-9280-2.

13 *and chronic stress can all lead to inflammation.*
Nicolas Rohleder, "Stress and Inflammation—The Need to Address the Gap in the Transition between Acute and Chronic Stress Effects," *Psychoneuroendocrinology* 105 (2019): 164–71, https://doi.org/10.1016/j.psyneuen.2019.02.021.

13 *Inflammation impacts the sleep centers of the brain and shortens the sleep cycles necessary for growth and repair.*
Irwin, Michael R. "Sleep and Inflammation: Partners in Sickness and in Health." *Nature Reviews Immunology* 19, no. 11 (2019): 702–715, https://doi.org/10.1038/s41577-019-0190-z.

CAUSES OF INFLAMMATION: NEUROLOGY & INFLAMMATION

13 *Head trauma*
Robert J. MacKay, "Brain Injury after Head Trauma: Pathophysiology, Diagnosis, and Treatment," *Veterinary Clinics of North America: Equine Practice* 20, no. 1 (2004): 199–216, https://doi.org/10.1016/j.cveq.2003.11.006.

13 *addiction to drugs*
Karen D. Ersche and Rainer Döffinger, "Inflammation and Infection in Human Cocaine Addiction," *Current Opinion in Behavioral Sciences* 13 (2017): 203–9, https://doi.org/10.1016/j.cobeha.2016.12.007.

13 *and too much light from screen time can all cause brain inflammation.*
Emmanuel Stamatakis, Mark Hamer, and David W. Dunstan, "Screen-Based Entertainment Time, All-Cause Mortality, and Cardiovascular Events: Population-Based Study with Ongoing Mortality and Hospital Events Follow-Up," *Journal of the American College of Cardiology* 57, no. 3 (January 2011): 292–99, https://doi.org/10.1016/j.jacc.2010.05.065.

14 *Other common causes for neurological inflammation include food intolerances*
Yoshikazu Ohtsuka, "Food Intolerance and Mucosal Inflammation," *Pediatrics International* 57, no. 1 (2015): 22–29, https://doi.org/10.1111/ped.12546.

CAUSES OF INFLAMMATION: EMOTIONAL CAUSES OF INFLAMMATION

15 *Abuse, neglect, grief, and other childhood traumas can unfortunately become a lifelong "operating system" that triggers ongoing inflammation.*
Mingyi Chen and Rebecca E. Lacey, "Adverse Childhood Experiences and Adult Inflammation: Findings from the 1958 British Birth Cohort," *Brain, Behavior, and Immunity* 69 (2018): 582–90, https://doi.org/10.1016/j.bbi.2018.02.007; Hartej Gill et al., "The Association between Adverse Childhood Experiences and Inflammation in Patients with Major Depressive Disorder: A Systematic Review," *Journal of Affective Disorders* 272 (2020): 1–7, https://doi.org/10.1016/j.jad.2020.03.145.

15 *Many therapeutic methods have been shown to help heal these traumas: meditation*
Carlo Dal Lin et al., "Toward a Unified View of Cognitive and Biochemical Activity: Meditation and Linguistic Self-Reconstructing May Lead to Inflammation and Oxidative Stress Improvement," *Entropy* 22, no. 8 (2020): 818, https://doi.org/ 10.3390/e22080818.

15 *mindfulness practices*
Stephanie Fountain-Zaragoza and Ruchika Shaurya Prakash, "Mindfulness Training for Healthy Aging: Impact on Attention, Well-Being, and Inflammation," *Frontiers in Aging Neuroscience* 9 (2017): 11, https://doi.org/10.3389/fnagi.2017.00011.

15 *neurofeedback, EMDR therapy (eye movement desensitization and reprocessing)*
Sara Carletto et al., "Treating Post-Traumatic Stress Disorder in Patients with Multiple Sclerosis: A Randomized Controlled Trial Comparing the Efficacy of Eye Movement Desensitization and Reprocessing and Relaxation Therapy," *Frontiers in Psychology* 7 (21 April 2016): 526, https://doi.org/10.3389/fpsyg.2016.00526.

15 *cognitive therapy*
Adrian L. Lopresti, "Cognitive Behaviour Therapy and Inflammation: A Systematic Review of Its Relationship and the Potential Implications for the Treatment of Depression," *The Australian and New Zealand Journal of Psychiatry* 51, no. 6 (2017): 565–82, https://doi.org/10.1177/0004867417701996.

15 *EFT (emotional freedom technique, or tapping)*
Wendy L. Waite and Mark D. Holder, "Assessment of the Emotional Freedom Technique," *Scientific Review of Mental Health Practice* 2, no. 1 (2003): 1–10, https://www.srmhp.org/0201/emotional-freedom-technique.html.

15 *Additionally, psilocybin-guided therapy*
Susan Ling et al., "Molecular Mechanisms of Psilocybin and Implications for the Treatment of Depression," *CNS Drugs* 36, no. 1 (January 2022): 17–30, https://doi.org/10.1007/s40263-021-00877-y; Drummond E-Wen McCulloch et al., "Lasting Effects of a Single Psilocybin Dose on Resting-State Functional Connectivity in Healthy Individuals," *Journal of Psychopharmacology* 36, no. 1 (January 2022): 74–84, , https://doi.org/10.1177/02698811211026454.

15 *ketamine treatments*
Ronald S. Duman, "Ketamine and Rapid-Acting Antidepressants: A New Era in the Battle against Depression and Suicide," *F1000Research*

7 (May 24, 2018): Faculty Rev-659, https://doi.org/10.12688/f1000research.14344.1; Roger S. McIntyre et al., "Synthesizing the Evidence for Ketamine and Esketamine in Treatment-Resistant Depression: An International Expert Opinion on the Available Evidence and Implementation," *American Journal of Psychiatry* 178, no. 5 (May 1, 2021): 383–99, https://doi.org/10.1176/appi.ajp.2020.20081251; Thu Ha Pham and Alain M. Gardier, "Fast-Acting Antidepressant Activity of Ketamine: Highlights on Brain Serotonin, Glutamate, and GABA Neurotransmission in Preclinical Studies," *Pharmacology & Therapeutics* 199 (July 2019): 58–90, https://doi.org/10.1016/j.pharmthera.2019.02.017.

15 *and ayahuasca treatments . . . have been shown to improve neural pathways.*
Marina Goulart da Silva, Guilherme Cabreira Daros, and Rafael Mariano de Bitencourt, "Anti-Inflammatory Activity of Ayahuasca: Therapeutical Implications in Neurological and Psychiatric Diseases," *Behavioural Brain Research* 400 (February 2021): 113003, https://doi.org/10.1016/j.bbr.2020.113003; Ede Frecska, Petra Bokor, and Michael Winkelman, "The Therapeutic Potentials of Ayahuasca: Possible Effects against Various Diseases of Civilization," *Frontiers in Pharmacology* 7 (March 2, 2016): 35, https://doi.org/10.3389/fphar.2016.00035; Jonathan Hamill et al., "Ayahuasca: Psychological and Physiologic Effects, Pharmacology and Potential Uses in Addiction and Mental Illness," *Current Neuropharmacology* 17, no. 2 (January 7, 2019): 108–28, https://doi.org/10.2174/1570159X16666180125095902.

CAUSES OF INFLAMMATION: CORTISOL, ESTROGEN, INSULIN & INFLAMMATION

15 *People with chronic inflammation often have cortisol levels that are chronically high or low, though high is more common.*
Tawfiq Almadi, Ian Cathers, and Chin Moi Chow, "Associations among Work-Related Stress, Cortisol, Inflammation, and Metabolic Syndrome," *Psychophysiology* 50, no. 9 (2013): 821–30, https://doi.org/10.1111/psyp.12069.

15 *When your cortisol levels are off, they can trigger autoimmune disorders*
M. Neidhart, "Elevated Serum Prolactin or Elevated Prolactin/Cortisol Ratio Are Associated with Autoimmune Processes in Systemic Lupus

Erythematosus and Other Connective Tissue Diseases," *The Journal of Rheumatology* 23, no. 3 (1996): 476–81, https://pubmed.ncbi.nlm.nih.gov/8832986/.

15 *along with food and chemical intolerances.*
Aziz Koleilat, "Food Intolerance," *Biomedical Journal of Scientific & Technical Research* 1, no. 2 (July 2017), https://doi.org/10.26717/BJSTR.2017.01.000190.

16 *[Imbalanced cortisol levels] can also disrupt reproductive hormones*
C. R. Ralph et al., "Impact of Psychosocial Stress on Gonadotrophins and Sexual Behaviour in Females: Role for Cortisol?" *Reproduction* 152, no. 1 (2016): R1–14, https://doi.org/10.1530/REP-15-0604.

16 *and thyroid hormone activity.*
Yoichi Ichikawa et al., "Altered Equilibrium between Cortisol and Cortisone in Plasma in Thyroid Dysfunction and Inflammatory Diseases," *Metabolism* 26, no. 9 (1977): 989–97.

16 *Furthermore, chronically high cortisol induces intestinal permeability (leaky gut)*
John W. Cartmell, "Cortisol and Diabetes," *Townsend Letter: The Examiner of Alternative Medicine*, no. 280 (2006): 114–16; Ye Zong et al., "Chronic Stress and Intestinal Permeability: Lubiprostone Regulates Glucocorticoid Receptor-Mediated Changes in Colon Epithelial Tight Junction Proteins, Barrier Function, and Visceral Pain in the Rodent and Human," *Neurogastroenterology and Motility* 31, no. 2 (February 2019): e13477, https://doi.org/10.1111/nmo.13477.

16 *which causes more food intolerances, digestive problems, and intestinal inflammation.*
Ricard Farré et al., "Intestinal Permeability, Inflammation and the Role of Nutrients," *Nutrients* 12, no. 4 (April 23, 2020): 1185, https://doi.org/10.3390/nu12041185.

16 *Cortisol imbalances are brought on by chronic stress.*
Do Yup Lee, Eosu Kim, and Man Ho Choi, "Technical and Clinical Aspects of Cortisol as a Biochemical Marker of Chronic Stress," *BMB Reports* 48, no. 4 (2015): 209–16; https://doi.org/10.5483/bmbrep.2015.48.4.275.

ENDNOTES

16 *When estrogen levels are off—whether estrogen is too high, too low, or, worst of all, constantly fluctuating as it does during perimenopause—women may experience inflammatory issues and other challenges.*
Subhadeep Chakrabarti, Olga Lekontseva, and Sandra T. Davidge, "Estrogen Is a Modulator of Vascular Inflammation," *IUBMB Life* 60, no. 6 (2008): 376–82; https://doi.org/10.1002/iub.48.

16 *Symptoms of hormonal imbalances in women include irregular cycles, PMS*
Torbjörn Bäckström, et al., "The Role of Hormones and Hormonal Treatments in Premenstrual Syndrome," *CNS Drugs* 17, no. 5 (2003): 325–342, https://doi.org/10.2165/00023210-200317050-00003; Suhail A. R. Doi, et al., "Irregular Cycles and Steroid Hormones in Polycystic Ovary Syndrome," Human Reproduction 20, no. 9 (2005): 2402–2408, https://doi.org/10.1093/humrep/dei093.

16 *infertility*
Kathiuska J. Kriedt, Ali Alchami, and Melanie C. Davies, "PCOS: Diagnosis and Management of Related Infertility," *Obstetrics, Gynaecology & Reproductive Medicine* 29, no. 1 (2019): 1–5, https://doi.org/10.1016/j.ogrm.2018.12.001.

16 *PCOS*
Antoni J. Duleba and Anuja Dokras, "Is PCOS an Inflammatory Process?," *Fertility and Sterility* 97, no. 1 (2012): 7–12, https://doi.org/10.1016/j.fertnstert.2011.11.023; Ewa Rudnicka et al., "Chronic Low Grade Inflammation in Pathogenesis of PCOS," *International Journal of Molecular Sciences* 22, no. 7 (2021): 3789, https://doi.org/10.3390/ijms22073789.

16 *and a difficult time transitioning into menopause.*
Sabahat Rasool and Duru Shah, "Polycystic Ovary Syndrome (PCOS) Transition at Menopause," *Journal of Mid-Life Health* 12, no. 1 (2021): 30–32, https://doi.org/10.4103/jmh.jmh_37_21.

17 *Insulin is a hormone that helps regulate blood sugar by escorting glucose into cells to be used for energy.*
Gisela Wilcox, "Insulin and Insulin Resistance," *Clinical Biochemist Reviews* 26, no. 2 (2005): 19–39, https://pubmed.ncbi.nlm.nih.gov/16278749/.

17 *Insulin resistance is a big issue for inflammation.*
Carl de Luca and Jerrold M. Olefsky, "Inflammation and Insulin Resistance," *FEBS Letters* 582, no. 1 (2008): 97–105, https://doi.org/10.1016/j.febslet.2007.11.057.

17 *Aside from high blood sugar, the most common signs of insulin resistance are excess belly fat, feeling sleepy after meals, and poor sleep.*
Wilcox, "Insulin and Insulin Resistance," 19–39.

ENVIRONMENTAL TOXINS & HOW TO BUFFER THEM

18 *Multiple studies show people carry toxins in their bodies*
Erin Jackson et al., "Adipose Tissue as a Site of Toxin Accumulation," *Comprehensive Physiology* 7, no. 4 (2017): 1085–1135, https://doi.org/10.1002/cphy.c160038.

18 *[toxins] have been found in breast milk*
Kadriye Yurdakök, "Lead, Mercury, and Cadmium in Breast Milk," *Journal of Pediatric and Neonatal Individualized Medicine (JPNIM)* 4, no. 2 (2015): e040223–e040223, https://doi.org/10.7363/040223.

18 *and even fetal placenta cords.*
Go Suzuki, Masuo Nakano, and Shiro Nakano, "Distribution of PCDDs/PCDFs and Co-PCBs in Human Maternal Blood, Cord Blood, Placenta, Milk, and Adipose Tissue: Dioxins Showing High Toxic Equivalency Factor Accumulate in the Placenta," *Bioscience, Biotechnology, and Biochemistry* 69, no. 10 (2005): 1836–47, https://doi.org/10.1271/bbb.69.1836.

18 *Endocrine disruptors are chemicals that disrupt how our hormones function by mimicking the structure of natural hormones, confusing the body, or altering how hormones function.*
Cristina Casals-Casas and Béatrice Desvergne, "Endocrine Disruptors: From Endocrine to Metabolic Disruption," *Annual Review of Physiology* 73 (2011): 135–62, https://doi.org/10.1146/annurev-physiol-012110-142200.

ENDNOTES

ENVIRONMENTAL TOXINS & HOW TO BUFFER THEM: BPA & BPS

19   *BPS was the replacement chemical for BPA in products that are BPA-free, but it is more potent in terms of hazard.*
Soria Eladak et al., "A New Chapter in the Bisphenol A Story: Bisphenol S and Bisphenol F Are Not Safe Alternatives to This Compound," *Fertility and Sterility* 103, no. 1 (2015): 11–21, https://doi.org/10.1016/j.fertnstert.2014.11.005; Melissa Ferguson, Ilka Lorenzen-Schmidt, and W. Glen Pyle, "Bisphenol S Rapidly Depresses Heart Function through Estrogen Receptor-β and Decreases Phospholamban Phosphorylation in a Sex-Dependent Manner," *Scientific Reports* 9, no. 1 (2019): 15948, https://doi.org/10.1038/s41598-019-52350-y.

19   *According to government tests, 93% of Americans have BPA in their bodies*
Iris Corbasson et al., "Urinary Bisphenol-A, Phthalate Metabolites and Body Composition in US Adults, NHANES 1999–2006," *International Journal of Environmental Health Research* 26, no. 5–6 (2016): 606–17, https://doi.org/10.1080/09603123.2016.1233524.

19   *a separate study in 2015–2016 found 97% of participants had BPA in their urine samples.*
Melanie H. Jacobson et al., "Urinary Bisphenols and Obesity Prevalence among U.S. Children and Adolescents," *Journal of the Endocrine Society* 3, no. 9 (2019): 1715–26, https://doi.org/10.1210/js.2019-00201.

19   *Compared to bodies that have none, bodies with BPA in urine have a 21% increase in inflammatory markers.*
Deborah J. Watkins et al., "Associations between Urinary Phenol and Paraben Concentrations and Markers of Oxidative Stress and Inflammation among Pregnant Women in Puerto Rico," *International Journal of Hygiene and Environmental Health* 218, no. 2 (March 2015): 212–19, https://doi.org/10.1016/j.ijheh.2014.11.001.

THE INFLAMMATORY RESET

ENVIRONMENTAL TOXINS & HOW TO BUFFER THEM: DIOXINS

20 *Dioxins are a group of chemicals that form, most often, from incomplete burning of household and industrial waste.*
Arnold Schecter et al., "Dioxins: An Overview," *Environmental Research* 101, no. 3 (2006): 419–28, https://doi.org/10.1016/j.envres.2005.12.003.

20 *Dioxins are well studied, and research shows that they are some of the most proinflammatory toxins in the environment, commonly inducing chronic inflammation in the body.*
Michael C. Petriello et al., "Dioxin-Like PCB 126 Increases Systemic Inflammation and Accelerates Atherosclerosis in Lean LDL Receptor-Deficient Mice," *Toxicological Sciences* 162, no. 2 (2018): 548–58, https://doi.org/10.1093/toxsci/kfx275.

20 *This immune activation directly influences male and female reproductive systems, lowering sperm quality and count in males and promoting endometriosis in females. In terms of reproduction, damage can start in utero when the fetus is exposed to even low levels of dioxins, which can disrupt hormone signaling and reproductive development.*
Sherry Rier and Warren G. Foster, "Environmental Dioxins and Endometriosis," *Toxicological Sciences* 70, no. 2 (2002): 161–70, https://doi.org/10.1093/toxsci/70.2.161.

ENVIRONMENTAL TOXINS & HOW TO BUFFER THEM: HOW TO AVOID DIOXINS

20 *Eat fewer animal-based products.*
George F. Fries, "A Review of the Significance of Animal Food Products as Potential Pathways of Human Exposures to Dioxins," *Journal of Animal Science* 73, no. 6 (1995): 1639–50, https://doi.org/10.2527/1995.7361639x.

20 *One study shows those who eat a plant-based diet have the least amount of dioxin exposure.*
Ann L. Yaktine, Gail G. Harrison, and Robert S. Lawrence, "Reducing Exposure to Dioxins and Related Compounds through Foods in the Next Generation," *Nutrition Reviews* 64, no. 9 (2006): 403–9, https://doi.org/10.1111/j.1753-4887.2006.tb00225.x.

ENDNOTES

ENVIRONMENTAL TOXINS & HOW TO BUFFER THEM: PARABENS

21 *Parabens—synthetic preservatives that extend shelf life, hinder the growth of bacteria—are used in a variety of products, including cosmetics, pharmaceuticals, and food.*
P. D. Darbre et al., "Concentrations of Parabens in Human Breast Tumours," *Journal of Applied Toxicology* 24, no. 1 (January 2004): 5–13, https://doi.org/10.1002/jat.958.

21 *Researchers have also found measurable amounts of parabens in some 90% of typical grocery items—such as beers, sauces, desserts, soft drinks, jams, pickles, frozen dairy products, processed vegetables, and flavoring syrups.*
Chunyang Liao, Fang Liu, and Kurunthachalam Kannan, "Occurrence of and Dietary Exposure to Parabens in Foodstuffs from the United States," *Environmental Science & Technology* 47, no. 8 (2013): 3918–25, https://doi.org/10.1021/es400724s.

21 *[they] can trigger inflammation, disrupt hormone balance, impact fertility and reproductive organs, and affect birth outcomes.*
Hilde Kristin Vindenes et al., "Exposure to Environmental Phenols and Parabens, and Relation to Body Mass Index, Eczema and Respiratory Outcomes in the Norwegian RHINESSA Study," *Environmental Health* 20, no. 1 (2021): 81, https://doi.org/10.1186/s12940-021-00767-2.

21 *One study detected traces of five parabens in the breast tumors of 19 out of 20 women.*
P. D. Darbre et al., "Concentrations of Parabens in Human Breast Tumours," *Journal of Applied Toxicology* 24, no. 1 (January 2004): 5–13, https://doi.org/10.1002/jat.958.

ENVIRONMENTAL TOXINS & HOW TO BUFFER THEM: PHTHALATES

22 *Known as "the everywhere chemical," phthalates are a group of chemicals that make plastics flexible and hard to break.*
Russ Hauser and A. M. Calafat, "Phthalates and Human Health,"

Occupational and Environmental Medicine 62, no. 11 (2005): 806–18, https://doi.org/10.1136/oem.2004.017590.

23 *Exposure to phthalates has been found to induce inflammation and cause an inflammatory response in the endocrine system.*
Luoyao Yang et al., "Seasonal Exposure to Phthalates and Inflammatory Parameters: A Pilot Study with Repeated Measures," *Ecotoxicology and Environmental Safety* 208 (January 2021): 111633, https://doi.org/10.1016/j.ecoenv.2020.111633.

23 *Phthalates are linked with altered development of genitals, low sperm count, and poor sperm quality.*
Julia R. Barrett, "Phthalates and Baby Boys: Potential Disruption of Human Genital Development," *Environmental Health Perspectives* 113, no. 8 (August 2005): A542, https://www.ncbi.nlm.nih.gov/pmc/articles/PMC1280383/.

23 *Phthalates also cross through the placenta.*
Yiyu Qian et al., "The Endocrine Disruption of Prenatal Phthalate Exposure in Mother and Offspring," *Frontiers in Public Health* 8 (August 2020): 366, https://doi.org/10.3389/fpubh.2020.00366.

ENVIRONMENTAL TOXINS & HOW TO BUFFER THEM: PFAS (PERFLUOROALKYL & POLYFLUOROALKYL SUBSTANCES)

24 *In fact, research shows that 99% of Americans have PFAS in their bodies.*
Kayoko Kato et al., "Trends in Exposure to Polyfluoroalkyl Chemicals in the US Population: 1999–2008," *Environmental Science & Technology* 45, no. 19 (2011): 8037–45, https://doi.org/10.1021/es1043613.

24 *Exposure to PFAS has been linked to decreased sperm quality, low birth weight, kidney disease, thyroid disease, and high cholesterol, among other health issues.*
Martyn Kirk et al., "The PFAS Health Study: Systematic Literature Review," (Canberra: National Centre for Epidemiology and Population Health, The Australian National University, 2018), https://doi.org/10.25911/KW6T-7H44.

ENDNOTES

ENVIRONMENTAL TOXINS & HOW TO BUFFER THEM: HOW TO AVOID PFAS

24 *Avoid Teflon or nonstick cookware. If you choose to continue using nonstick cookware, be careful not to let it heat above 450°F. Do not leave nonstick cookware unattended on the stove or use it in hot ovens or on grills. Use cast-iron, 100% ceramic, or high-quality stainless-steel cookware.*
Muhammad Sajid and Muhammad Ilyas, "PTFE-Coated Non-Stick Cookware and Toxicity Concerns: A Perspective," *Environmental Science and Pollution Research* 24, no. 30 (October 2017): 23436–40, https://doi.org/10.1007/s11356-017-0095-y.

ENVIRONMENTAL TOXINS & HOW TO BUFFER THEM: GLYPHOSATE

25 *Studies suggest even relatively low levels of glyphosate may be endocrine disruptors*
Céline Gasnier et al., "Glyphosate-Based Herbicides Are Toxic and Endocrine Disruptors in Human Cell Lines," *Toxicology* 262, no. 3 (August 2009): 184–91, https://doi.org/10.1016/j.tox.2009.06.006; John Peterson Myers et al., "Concerns over Use of Glyphosate-Based Herbicides and Risks Associated with Exposures: A Consensus Statement," *Environmental Health* 15 (December 2016): 19, https://doi.org/10.1186/s12940-016-0117-0.

25 *with the ability to potentially reduce testosterone levels*
Sunny O. Abarikwu et al., "Combined Effects of Repeated Administration of Bretmont Wipeout (Glyphosate) and Ultrazin (Atrazine) on Testosterone, Oxidative Stress and Sperm Quality of Wistar Rats," *Toxicology Mechanisms and Methods* 25, no. 1 (2015): 70–80, https://doi.org/10.3109/15376516.2014.989349; Émilie Clair et al., "A Glyphosate-Based Herbicide Induces Necrosis and Apoptosis in Mature Rat Testicular Cells in Vitro, and Testosterone Decrease at Lower Levels," *Toxicology in Vitro* 26, no. 2 (March 2012): 269–79, https://doi.org/10.1016/j.tiv.2011.12.009.

25 *impair sperm quality*
Abarikwu et al., "Combined Effects of Repeated Administration of Bretmont Wipeout (Glyphosate) and Ultrazin (Atrazine)," 70–80; Folarin O. Owagboriaye et al., "Reproductive Toxicity of Roundup Herbicide Exposure in Male Albino Rat," *Experimental and Toxicologic Pathology* 69, no. 7 (2017): 461–68, https://doi.org/10.1016/j.etp.2017.04.007.

25 *or cause disturbances in reproductive development.*
R. M. Romano et al., "Prepubertal Exposure to Commercial Formulation of the Herbicide Glyphosate Alters Testosterone Levels and Testicular Morphology," *Archives of Toxicology* 84, no. 4 (April 2010): 309–17, https://doi.org/10.1007/s00204-009-0494-z.

ENVIRONMENTAL TOXINS & HOW TO BUFFER THEM: FLAME RETARDANTS

26 *These powerful and toxic [flame retardants] are significant endocrine and thyroid disruptors that impact immune and reproductive function, raise the risk of cancer, and affect fetal and child development and neurologic functions.*
Lucio G. Costa et al., "Polybrominated Diphenyl Ether (PBDE) Flame Retardants: Environmental Contamination, Human Body Burden and Potential Adverse Health Effects," *Acta Biomedica: Atenei Parmensis* 79, no. 3 (2008): 172–83, https://pubmed.ncbi.nlm.nih.gov/19260376/; Young Ran Kim et al., "Health Consequences of Exposure to Brominated Flame Retardants: A Systematic Review," *Chemosphere* 106 (2014): 1–19, https://doi.org/10.1016/j.chemosphere.2013.12.064.

COVID LONG-HAULERS & INFLAMMATION

27 *Covid reacts with different tissues of the body*
Aristo Vojdani and Datis Kharrazian, "Potential antigenic cross-reactivity between SARS-CoV-2 and human tissue with a possible link to an increase in autoimmune diseases," *Clinical Immunology* 217 (2020): 108480. https://doi.org/10.1016/j.clim.2020.108480

ENDNOTES

ACTIVITIES & EXERCISES TO REDUCE INFLAMMATION: EXERCISE

34 *However, studies show daily physical activity helps manage symptoms from inflammation compared to not exercising at all.*
Ronenn Roubenoff, "Physical Activity, Inflammation, and Muscle Loss," *Nutrition Reviews* 65, no. suppl_3 (2007): S208–12, https://doi.org/10.1111/j.1753-4887.2007.tb00364.x.

34 *Additionally, people who engage in regular physical activity report less depression and better self-esteem and increased happiness.*
Robert F. Zoeller Jr., "Physical Activity: Depression, Anxiety, Physical Activity, and Cardiovascular Disease: What's the Connection?," *American Journal of Lifestyle Medicine* 1, no. 3 (2007): 175–80, https://doi.org/10.1177/1559827607300518.

34 *High-intensity interval training (HIIT), in particular, dilates blood vessels, lowers inflammation, and improves blood flow to the brain.*
Matthew Weston et al., "Effects of Low-Volume High-Intensity Interval Training (HIT) on Fitness in Adults: A Meta-Analysis of Controlled and Non-Controlled Trials," *Sports Medicine* 44, no. 7 (2014): 1005–17, https://doi.org/10.1007/s40279-014-0180-z.

35 *If someone has a severe autoimmune disease or a severe inflammatory condition, exercise initially may make things worse because it increases exercise-induced cytokines that create an inflammatory response and can exacerbate symptoms.*
Jonatas E. Nogueira et al., "Molecular Hydrogen Reduces Acute Exercise-Induced Inflammatory and Oxidative Stress Status," *Free Radical Biology and Medicine* 129 (December 2018): 186–93, https://doi.org/10.1016/j.freeradbiomed.2018.09.028.

ACTIVITIES & EXERCISES TO REDUCE INFLAMMATION: MEDITATION

35 *Meditation and other mindfulness practices can improve your emotional well-being and the health of your subconscious "operating system."*
Madhav Goyal et al., "Meditation Programs for Psychological Stress

and Well-Being: A Systematic Review and Meta-Analysis," *JAMA Internal Medicine* 174, no. 3 (2014): 357–68, https://doi.org/10.1001/jamainternmed.2013.13018.

ACTIVITIES & EXERCISES TO REDUCE INFLAMMATION: STIMULATING THE VAGUS NERVE

36 *Studies also show that stimulating the vagus nerve helps dampen inflammation and symptoms of autoimmune disorders.*
Robert H. Howland, "Vagus Nerve Stimulation," *Current Behavioral Neuroscience Reports* 1, no. 2 (June 2014): 64–73, https://doi.org/10.1007/s40473-014-0010-5.

ACTIVITIES & EXERCISES TO REDUCE INFLAMMATION: ICE BATHS & COLD SHOWERS

36 *Taking an ice bath or cold shower first thing in the morning will help stimulate the cortisol awakening response (CAR) and adrenal function to set the day off right.*
Nikolai A. Shevchuk, "Adapted Cold Shower as a Potential Treatment for Depression," *Medical Hypotheses* 70, no. 5 (January 2008): 995–1001, https://doi.org/10.1016/j.mehy.2007.04.052.

37 *two to three minutes in an ice bath in the morning or just one minute in a cold shower with deep breathing can stimulate an anti-inflammatory cholinergic pathway that will dampen inflammation.*
H. Hinkka et al., "Effects of Cold Mist Shower on Patients with Inflammatory Arthritis: A Crossover Controlled Clinical Trial," *Scandinavian Journal of Rheumatology* 46, no. 3 (2017): 206–9, https://doi.org/10.1080/03009742.2016.1199733.

ACTIVITIES & EXERCISES TO REDUCE INFLAMMATION: INFRARED SAUNA

37 *One of the most powerful tools for pain relief, detoxification, inflammation, and heart health is a far-infrared sauna.*
Joy N. Hussain et al., "Infrared Sauna as Exercise-Mimetic? Physiological Responses to Infrared Sauna vs Exercise in Healthy Women: A

Randomized Controlled Crossover Trial," *Complementary Therapies in Medicine* 64 (March 2022): 102798, https://doi.org/10.1016/j.ctim.2021.102798.

ACTIVITIES & EXERCISES TO REDUCE INFLAMMATION: ALPHA-STIM TRAINING

38 *Not only does the Alpha-Stim improve brain function, it also has been shown to relieve post-traumatic stress and acute and chronic pain.*
Richard Morriss et al., "Clinical Effectiveness and Cost Minimisation Model of Alpha-Stim Cranial Electrotherapy Stimulation in Treatment Seeking Patients with Moderate to Severe Generalised Anxiety Disorder," *Journal of Affective Disorders* 253 (2019): 426–37, https://doi.org/10.1016/j.jad.2019.04.020.

ACTIVITIES & EXERCISES TO REDUCE INFLAMMATION: HYPERBARIC OXYGEN THERAPY

38 *exponentially increasing the delivery of oxygen throughout your body and allowing it to reach inflamed tissues and infuse the body's cells for improved function.*
Patrick M. Tibbles and John S. Edelsberg, "Hyperbaric-Oxygen Therapy," *The New England Journal of Medicine* 334, no. 25 (1996): 1642–48, https://doi.org/10.1056/NEJM199606203342506.

SUPPLEMENTS & INFLAMMATION

43
Table *[Liposomal turmeric] dampens inflammation [and] improves integrity of the intestinal and blood-brain barriers.*
Arghavan Memarzia et al., "Experimental and Clinical Reports on Anti-inflammatory, Antioxidant, and Immunomodulatory Effects of Curcuma Longa and Curcumin, an Updated and Comprehensive Review," *BioFactors* 47, no. 3 (2021): 311–50, https://doi.org/10.1002/biof.1716.

43
Table *[Liposomal turmeric] should contain black pepper to enhance bioavailability and absorption.*

Zuzanna Bober et al., "Medicinal Benefits from the Use of Black Pepper, Curcuma and Ginger," *European Journal of Clinical and Experimental Medicine* 16, no. 2 (2018): 133–45, https://doi.org/10.15584/ejcem.2018. 2.9.

43 Table *[Liposomal resveratrol] dampens inflammation.*
Abeer M. Alanazi et al., "Liposomal Resveratrol and/or Carvedilol Attenuate Doxorubicin-Induced Cardiotoxicity by Modulating Inflammation, Oxidative Stress and S100A1 in Rats," *Antioxidants* 9, no. 2 (2020): 159, https://doi.org/10.3390/antiox9020159.

43 Table *[Vitamin D] supplements your vitamin D levels, which inflammation inhibits.*
Meg Mangin, Rebecca Sinha, and Kelly Fincher, "Inflammation and Vitamin D: The Infection Connection," *Inflammation Research* 63, no. 10 (2014): 803–19, https://doi.org/10.1007/s00011-014-0755-z.

44 Table *[Glutathione] protects brain and body cells from inflammatory damage.*
Frank J. Giblin, "Glutathione: A Vital Lens Antioxidant," *Journal of Ocular Pharmacology and Therapeutics* 16, no. 2 (2000): 121–35, https://doi.org/10.1089/jop.2000.16.121.

44 *Vitamin D is a negative acute phase reactant, which is a very technical way of saying that under inflammation, vitamin D decreases.*
Xavier Guillot et al., "Vitamin D and Inflammation," *Joint Bone Spine* 77, no. 6 (December 2010): 552–57, https://doi.org/10.1016/j.jbspin.2010.09.018.

44 *Vitamin D helps increase the amount of regulatory T cells (Tregs) that, as their name implies, regulate T cell proliferation.*
Martin Kongsbak et al., "The Vitamin D Receptor and T Cell Function," *Frontiers in Immunology* 4 (2013): 148, https://doi.org/10.3389/fimmu.2013.00148.

44 *When your body is confronted with dangerous bacteria or viruses in your body, T cells flourish to combat the infection in an autoimmune response.*

Steven Z. Josefowicz, Li-Fan Lu, and Alexander Y. Rudensky, "Regulatory T Cells: Mechanisms of Differentiation and Function," *Annual Review of Immunology* 30 (April 2012): 531–64, https://doi.org/10.1146/annurev.immunol.25.022106.141623.

45 *CBD and cannabis can potentially help with conditions such as epilepsy, arthritis, autoimmunity, Parkinson's, anxiety, depression, mood, inflammation, and so much more.*
Sumner Burstein, "Cannabidiol (CBD) and Its Analogs: A Review of Their Effects on Inflammation," *Bioorganic & Medicinal Chemistry* 23, no. 7 (2015): 1377–85, https://doi.org/10.1016/j.bmc.2015.01.059; C. Michael White, "A Review of Human Studies Assessing Cannabidiol's (CBD) Therapeutic Actions and Potential," *Journal of Clinical Pharmacology* 59, no. 7 (July 2019): 923–34, https://doi.org/10.1002/jcph.1387.

45 *Some people may have an allergic reaction or intolerance to the Cannabaceae family of flowering plants.*
Ine Ilona Decuyper et al., "Cannabis Allergy: What the Clinician Needs to Know in 2019," *Expert Review of Clinical Immunology* 15, no. 6 (2019): 599–606, https://doi.org/10.1080/1744666X.2019.1600403.

45 *Some marijuana strains stimulate inflammatory T cells, exacerbating an autoimmune response.*
Barbara L. F. Kaplan, Alison E. B. Springs, and Norbert E. Kaminski, "The Profile of Immune Modulation by Cannabidiol (CBD) Involves Deregulation of Nuclear Factor of Activated T Cells (NFAT)," *Biochemical Pharmacology* 76, no. 6 (2008): 726–37, https://doi.org/10.1016/j.bcp.2008.06.022.

FASTING WHILE ON THE INFLAMMATORY RESET: THE BENEFITS OF FASTING WITH INFLAMMATION

47 *Research shows fasting can quickly and dramatically lower inflammation and improve your immune, gut, and brain health.*
Valter D. Longo and Mark P. Mattson, "Fasting: Molecular Mechanisms and Clinical Applications," *Cell Metabolism* 19, no. 2 (2014): 181–92, https://doi.org/10.1016/j.cmet.2013.12.008.

47 *Including periods of fasting into your daily routine has been shown to help cells become more insulin sensitive, which in turn dampens the inflammation, metabolic imbalances, and brain degeneration caused by insulin resistance.*
Mark P. Mattson and Ruiqian Wan, "Beneficial Effects of Intermittent Fasting and Caloric Restriction on the Cardiovascular and Cerebrovascular Systems," *The Journal of Nutritional Biochemistry* 16, no. 3 (2005): 129–37, https://doi.org/10.1016/j.jnutbio.2004.12.007

47 *One study found restricting eating to a window of only eight hours each day significantly improved insulin resistance.*
Terra G. Arnason, Matthew W. Bowen, Kerry D. Mansell, "Effects of intermittent fasting on health markers in those with type 2 diabetes: A pilot study," *World Journal of Diabetes* 8, no. 4 (2017):154–164. https://doi.org/10.4239/wjd.v8.i4.154

47 *Intermittent fasting (for 12–18 hours each day) has been shown to improve immune function by reducing inflammation and minimizing the damage from inflammation.*
Mo'ez Al-Islam E. Faris et al., "Intermittent Fasting during Ramadan Attenuates Proinflammatory Cytokines and Immune Cells in Healthy Subjects," *Nutrition Research* 32, no. 12 (2012): 947–55, https://doi.org/10.1016/j.nutres.2012.06.021.

47 *[Intermittent fasting] also regulates immune function—great for autoimmune diseases—while also regenerating immune cells and even lowering the risk of cancer.*
Sebastian Brandhorst et al., "A Periodic Diet That Mimics Fasting Promotes Multi-System Regeneration, Enhanced Cognitive Performance, and Healthspan," *Cell Metabolism* 22, no. 1 (2015): 86–99, https://doi.org/10.1016/j.cmet.2015.05.012; Ayse L. Mindikoglu et al., "Intermittent Fasting from Dawn to Sunset for 30 Consecutive Days Is Associated with Anticancer Proteomic Signature and Upregulates Key Regulatory Proteins of Glucose and Lipid Metabolism, Circadian Clock, DNA Repair, Cytoskeleton Remodeling, Immune System and Cognitive Function in Healthy Subjects," *Journal of Proteomics* 217 (2020): 103645, https://doi.org/10.1016/j.jprot.2020.103645.

ENDNOTES

48 *[Fasting] supports autophagy*
Fernanda Antunes et al., "Autophagy and Intermittent Fasting: The Connection for Cancer Therapy?," *Clinics* 73, suppl 1 (2018): e814s, https://doi.org/10.6061/clinics/2018/e814s.

48 *Additionally, fasting boosts a brain chemical called brain-derived neurotrophic factor (BDNF), which protects your brain from neurodegenerative diseases such as Alzheimer's and Parkinson's.*
Basem H. Elesawy et al., "The Impact of Intermittent Fasting on Brain-Derived Neurotrophic Factor, Neurotrophin 3, and Rat Behavior in a Rat Model of Type 2 Diabetes Mellitus," *Brain Sciences* 11, no. 2 (2021): 242, https://doi.org/10.3390/brainsci11020242.

48 *Regular fasting can decrease "bad" cholesterol.*
Haiyan Meng et al., "Effects of Intermittent Fasting and Energy-Restricted Diets on Lipid Profile: A Systematic Review and Meta-Analysis," *Nutrition* 77 (2020): 110801, https://doi.org/10.1016/j.nut.2020.110801.

48 *Fasting has been shown to lower inflammation in the gut and create a healthier composition of gut bacteria.*
James H. Catterson et al., "Short-Term, Intermittent Fasting Induces Long-Lasting Gut Health and TOR-Independent Lifespan Extension," *Current Biology* 28, no. 11 (2018): 1714–24.e4, https://doi.org/10.1016/j.cub.2018.04.015.

ABOUT THE AUTHORS

DR. JOSH REDD has a total of 12 years of post-graduate education in health care, including two master's degrees and two doctorate degrees. He recently graduated from naturopathic medical school and is in the process of completing his residency. In addition to his naturopathic medical training, Dr. Redd has an MS in Human Nutrition and Functional Medicine and a MAPHB from Johns Hopkins with a graduating thesis titled "Underlying Mechanisms Driving Hashimoto's." In 2010, he graduated from Parker University with a Doctor of Chiropractic.

He is the founder of RedRiver Health and Wellness, one of the largest functional medicine clinics in the United States with eight practices in Utah, Arizona, New Mexico, Nevada, and Idaho. RedRiver treats patients from around the world who suffer from challenging thyroid disorders, Hashimoto's disease, and other autoimmune conditions.

Because the RedRiver practices treat hundreds of patients daily, Dr. Redd is able to identify patterns and trends among his patient population, as well as which evidence-based clinical strategies are the most successful in managing autoimmunity.

Dr. Redd is an Amazon #1 bestselling author and a published research biologist. He trains closely with Dr. Datis Kharrazian, PhD, DHSc, DC, MS, MMSc, FACN, Harvard Medical School Research Fellow, and Dr. Aristo Vojdani, PhD, MSc, and credits them for much of his success throughout the last 10 years as a functional medicine practitioner.

He delivers post-graduate lectures to health care professionals around the country on functional medicine topics such as neuroendocrine immunology, gastrointestinal disorders, gluten sensitivity and celiac disease, autoimmune management, functional blood chemistry, and clinical strategies for hypothyroidism and Hashimoto's.

ABOUT THE AUTHORS

Dr. Redd is passionate about his work managing the care of a growing number of professional athletes from around the world, including those in the NFL, MLB, NBA, and professional soccer in the US and Europe. He helps them create medical plans for diet, nutrition, strength training, recovery, and for necessary medical interventions when injured.

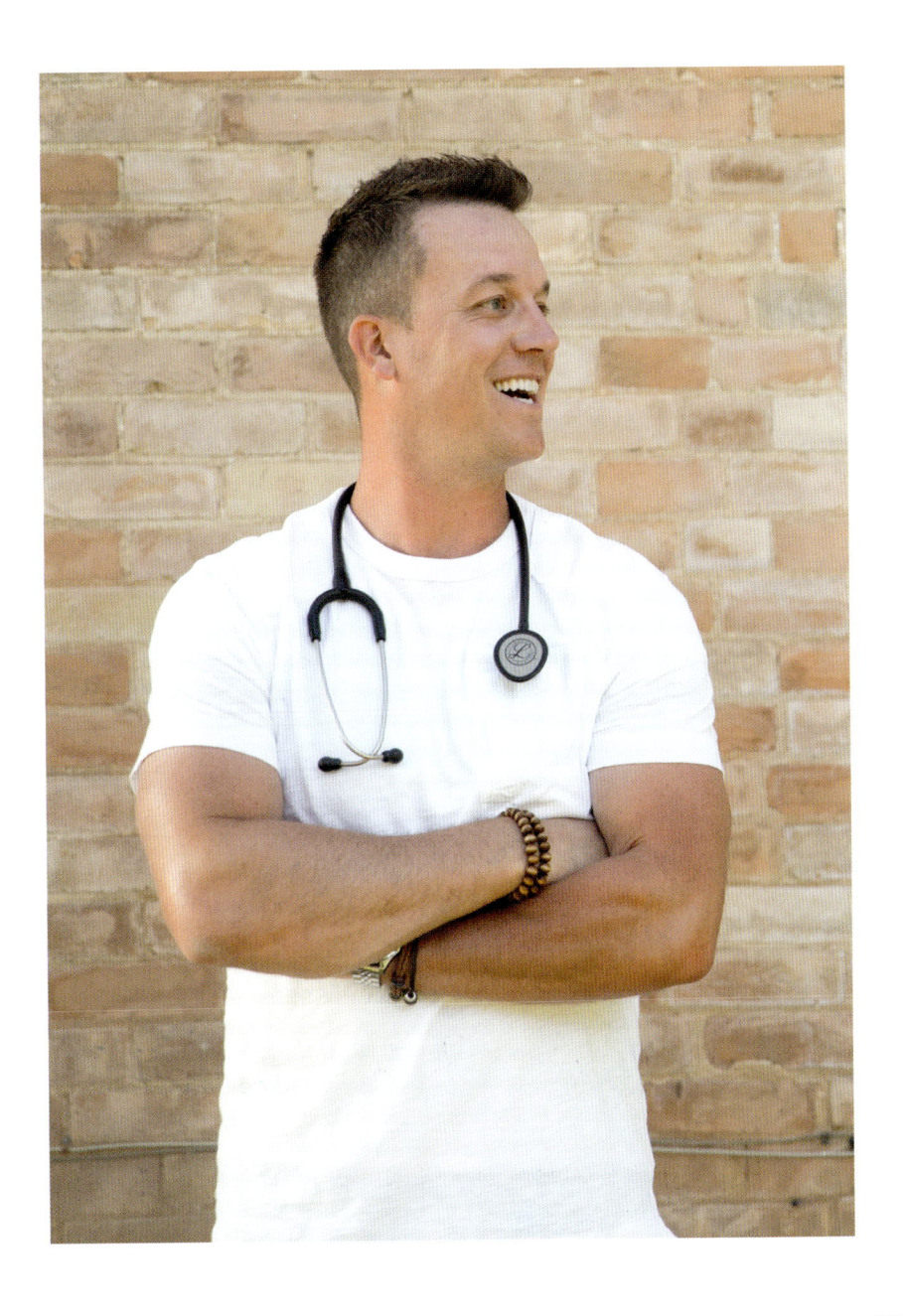

KARALYNNE CALL, Certified Nutritionist, is the founder of Just Ingredients, a health and wellness company dedicated to inspiring people to live happier, healthier lives. In a world where so many products contain so many hidden chemicals, Karalynne created the Just Ingredients product line to provide nourishing and natural options without sacrificing taste or effectiveness. Since the successful launch of her natural deodorant and organic face serum in 2019, Just Ingredients now sells over 16 different types of products, including their best-selling protein powders. Karalynne's vision to provide products made with natural ingredients was born out of her battle with severe depression. In this struggle, her life truly became a testament to the belief that nature provides exactly what we need to heal. Her passion for mental health and educating others on how to live a healthy life continues to inspire millions.

A mom of six, Karalynne began her wellness journey while working to heal entirely from depression. After years of doctor visits, medications, and a failed suicide attempt, she finally met a doctor who told her she could permanently heal from depression by eliminating toxins from her diet and daily use. Making this commitment truly saved Karalynne's life and transformed her family's future. She has made it her life's work to share her journey with others in hopes of inspiring people around the world to begin their own health journey.

Since then, Karalynne has grown her Instagram community, @Just.Ingredients, to nearly 1 million people. Her chart-topping podcast *Just Ingredients* has been host to nationally renowned experts and doctors who help her share the best ingredients for life. Having transformed countless lives and inspired a multitude of health journeys, Karalynne's impact and the Just Ingredients product line continues to grow exponentially by the day.

ABOUT THE AUTHORS

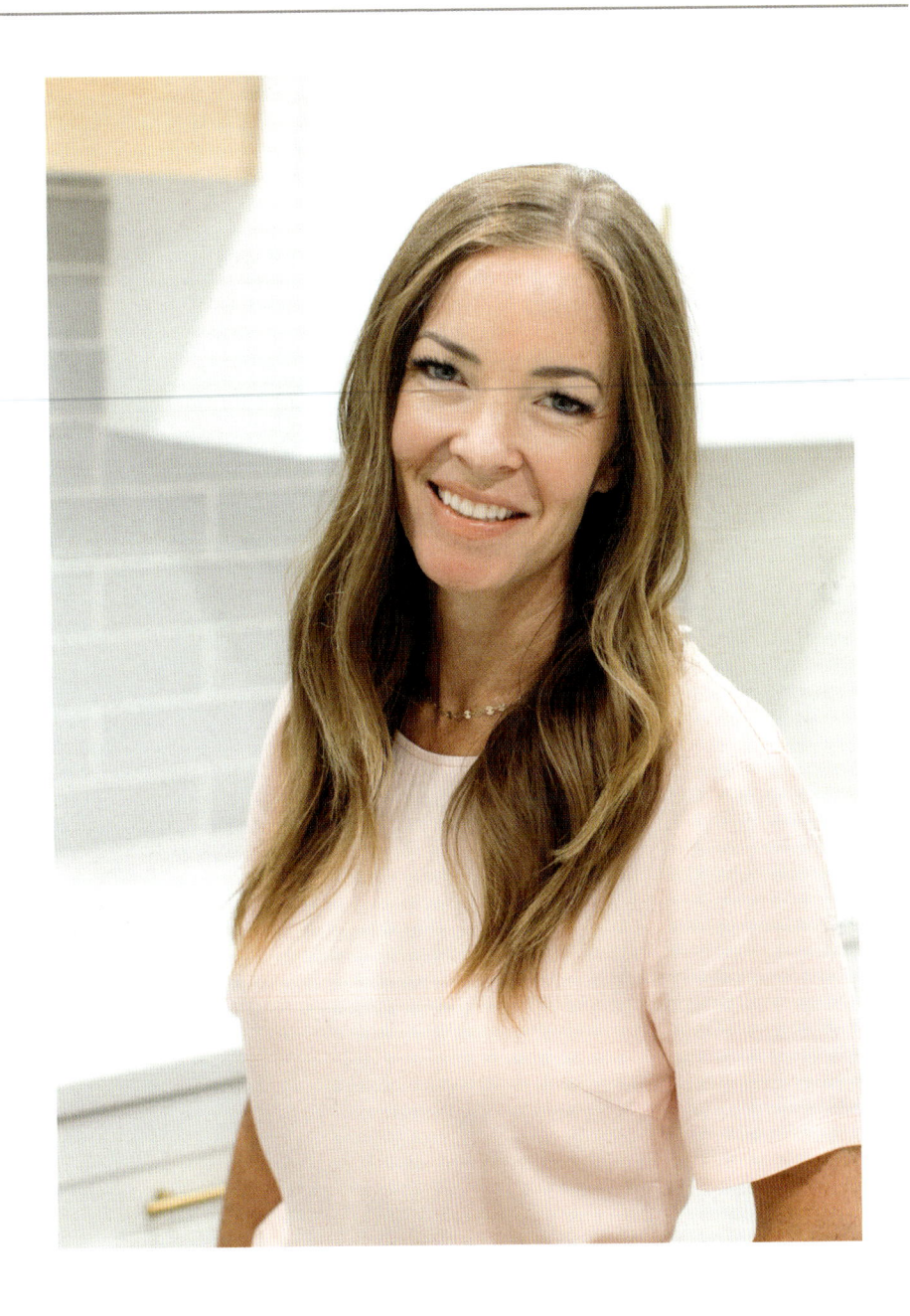

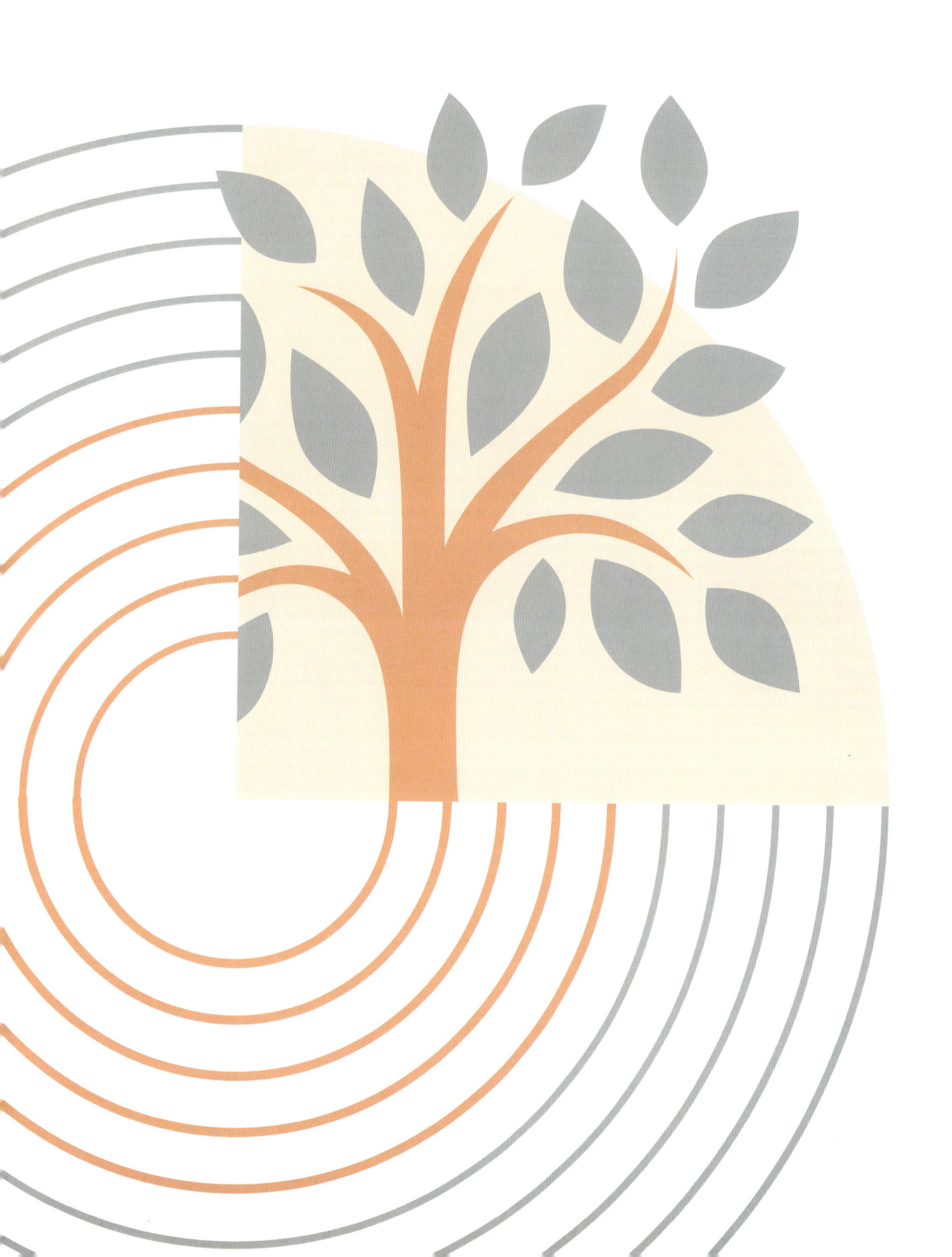